DEMENTIA SUPPORT FOR CAREGIVERS AND FAMILIES

Find Joy in Daily Care With Tools to Reduce Stress, Improve Communication and Nurture the Caregiver Bond

HANNA WELLS

Contents

Acknowledgments

First and foremost, I extend my heartfelt gratitude to all caregivers worldwide. Your unwavering commitment, patience, and compassion in providing care to those affected by dementia do not go unnoticed. Your ability to find strength in the face of adversity, to adapt and overcome, and to do so with love and dedication, is truly inspiring. This book is dedicated to you, in recognition of your invaluable role and the difference you make every day.

I express my profound appreciation to my family. Your support, encouragement, and understanding have been my anchor and source of strength. Your belief in the importance of this work has fueled my determination and passion. Thank you for standing by me, and with me, and for the love and laughter that kept me going during the most challenging times.

I also want to thank the special group of friends who listened, made suggestions, gave insights, and read and reread to help me make this work valuable to those who need it.

A special word of thanks goes to Jo Huey. Jo, your pioneering work, especially the "Ten Absolutes" (@Huey, 1996), has been instrumental in shaping the approach and content of this book. Your permission to incorporate the "Ten Absolutes" into this work is an honor, and I am deeply grateful for your generosity and support. Your contributions to the field of Alzheimer's and dementia care continue to inspire and guide caregivers and professionals alike.

In closing, I hope this book serves as a beacon of hope and a practical guide for caregivers and families. May it bring you comfort, increase your understanding, and help you find joy and fulfillment in your caregiving journey. Together, we can make a difference in the lives of those we care for and, in each other's lives, as we navigate this path with love, patience, and resilience.

Thank you all for being a part of this journey.

Hanna

Introduction

In the quiet spaces of our lives, where the routine once hummed with familiarity, a moment stops us in our tracks. It is a moment when the word "dementia" enters our world, rewriting the script of our lives without warning. Jennette Zarko, a compassionate wife navigating the challenging landscape of dementia, emotionally expressed the heart-wrenching truth: "When a loved one is diagnosed with dementia, you're left without a road map" (Zarko, 2018).

Meet Edgar, who faithfully protects his wife in the caregiving labyrinth through dementia. As her primary caregiver for a decade, he admits to learning new things daily. Edgar's life changed when his wife fell and broke her femur and three vertebrae. Edgar learned a lot from her behavior while taking painkillers. After seeing opioids transform lives, he encouraged families to seek a second opinion before using them. Edgar's minimalist approach to drug use has stabilized his wife's life after those falls. His story shows the complexities of caregiving and each caregiver's unique challenges, but it also warns that support and healing require a vigilant eye and a compassionate heart (Allen, 2021).

In a journey like Jennette and Edgar's, where uncertainty appears like a heavy fog, we find ourselves grappling with emotions as overwhelming as they are unpredictable. It's a path that seems daunting, lonely, and filled with questions for which we desperately seek answers. This is the road you've found yourself on, and I'm here to tell you that you are not alone.

What compelled you to pick up this book was not just a desire for knowledge but a yearning for a lifeline, a connection to someone who understands your struggles intimately. You seek not just information, but a roadmap crafted with empathy, a path that acknowledges the uniqueness of your journey. We will discuss some life-changing ideas to bring joy to daily care, improve communication, and relieve caregivers' suffering.

C.A.R.E.S.S. Method

The C.A.R.E.S.S. Method is a six-step approach designed to transform your caregiving experience into a more manageable, enriching, and even joyful endeavor.

Step 1 - Comprehension:

Let's unravel the complexities of dementia together, including its various types, stages, symptoms, and progression. By comprehending the disease, we empower ourselves to navigate its twists and turns more effectively.

Step 2 - Adaptation:

Discover the art of adaptation, how to tailor your communication, refine behavior management strategies, and nurture empathy and patience as the disease inevitably advances. This step is about evolving with grace.

Step 3 - Resilience:

Build emotional resilience to withstand the stress and emotional burdens of caregiving. This section offers tools to fortify your spirit, allowing you to face each day with renewed strength.

Step 4 - Empowerment:

Explore strategies to empower yourself through legal and financial insights, giving you the confidence to make decisions that safeguard your loved one's well-being and your own.

Step 5 - Success for the Future:

Look ahead, focusing on long-term care options and end-of-life planning. This step ensures that your caregiving journey is about the present and preparation for the future.

Step 6 - Self-care and Support:

Finally, discover the importance of creating a support network of friends, family, and more to share the load, celebrate the victories, and bolster each other in times of need.

Ten Absolutes of Alzheimer's Care

As a seasoned caregiver and author, I have witnessed firsthand the transformative power of effective communication in enhancing the lives of those navigating the challenging terrain of dementia. This book will discuss "Ten Absolutes" (@Huey, 1996), principles that have proven invaluable in fostering understanding, trust, and joy in caregiver-patient relationships.

1. Never Argue, Instead Agree

I advocate never arguing with individuals with dementia, opting to agree and provide reassurance instead. Drawing from personal experiences, such as the story of a resident caught in the grip of sundowning, I showcase the calming effect of agreement on the patient. By prioritizing their peace of mind over strict truthfulness, caregivers can guide individuals through moments of confusion with empathy and understanding.

2. Never Reason, Instead Divert

Building on the importance of validation, the second step explores the strategy of diverting conversations rather than reasoning with patients. Through a poignant anecdote involving a gentleman battling Lewy Body Dementia, we learn how gently shifting the focus can defuse tense situations and foster trust. Caregivers can create a supportive environment that promotes a sense of security by engaging in light conversation and validating the patient's feelings.

3. Never Shame, Instead Distract

In the third point, I emphasize the significance of avoiding shame and employing distraction techniques. Through the story of a woman who found solace in pacing, we discover the effectiveness of compliments, visualization, and engaging in past interests to redirect focus. This part highlights the power of thoughtful distractions in alleviating anxiety and promoting a sense of calm.

4. Never Lecture, Instead Reassure

This portion underscores the value of reassurance over lecturing, showcasing the story of a distressed 90-year-old woman. By gently reassuring her and offering support, caregivers can ease anxieties and provide validation, fostering a more peaceful state of mind for the patient.

5. Never Say Remember, Instead Reminisce

I delve into the importance of engaging in conversations about long-term memories, emphasizing their impact on individuals with dementia. Through the touching story of a gentleman finding comfort in sharing his upbringing, readers will understand the significance of reminiscing as a tool for connection.

6. Never Say I Told You, Instead Repeat or Regroup

Point six explores the necessity of repetition without making patients feel incompetent. Through stories like Mary's, who prepared for a doctor's appointment with unique attire, caregivers learn the importance of patience and understanding when repeating information, preserving dignity while providing support.

7. Never Say You Can't, Instead Say Do What You Can

In the seventh piece of advice, I advocate for empowerment through choice, sharing stories of residents like Mary and an 85-year-old with a unique wish to get her ears pierced. By focusing on abilities and providing opportunities for decision-making, caregivers can enhance the sense of agency and joy for individuals with dementia.

8. Never Command or Demand, Instead Ask or Model

It highlights the importance of gentle and understanding approaches, using a narrative involving a lady and her collection of stuffed animals. Caregivers can navigate situations empathetically by asking and suggesting instead of demanding, creating a more harmonious caregiving environment.

9. Never Condescend, Instead Encourage and Praise

I stress the significance of encouraging and praising individuals with dementia. Through stories like the Easter Bunny incident, readers gain insights into the gentle and compassionate approaches that can foster a positive and trusting caregiver-patient relationship.

10. Never Force, Instead Reinforce

The final segment discusses the essential rules in caregiving, including adaptability, creativity, and empathy. Readers learn about the transformative power of creative and empathetic strategies in reinforcing the patient's sense of reality and identity through the story of a gentleman's periodic urge to go to work.

Benefits of Reading This Book

This book provides a holistic guide for navigating the complex journey of dementia caregiving, It underscores the emotional and psychological challenges patients and caregivers face, advocating for patience and empathy as solid foundational elements for effective care while focusing on personal growth and resilience.

It further offers an array of practical strategies for enhancing communication and behavior management depicted through real-life stories and personal narratives. By applying these strategies, caregivers can improve their effectiveness and deepen their emotional connection with their loved ones, making every moment count.

Advocating a balanced approach, where taking care of oneself is as important as caring for a loved one, the book emphasizes building strong support networks and practicing self-care to maintain physical and emotional well-being. This approach is vital for sustaining the demanding role of caregiving over time.

Essential guidance is provided on caregiving's complex legal and financial aspects, empowering caregivers with knowledge and confidence. From understanding rights and obligations to managing finances effectively, the book is a crucial guide in these critical areas to alleviate concerns and ensure informed decision-making.

By reading "Dementia Support for Caregivers and Families," caregivers will gain invaluable shortcuts to:

1. Understand the complexities of dementia and effectively manage the disease.
2. Improve communication strategies, foster stronger relationships, and reduce frustration.
3. Enhance caregiving skills for daily care and behavior management and cultivate empathy.
4. Develop emotional resilience to manage the stress and emotional burden of caregiving.
5. Learn legal and financial strategies to navigate the challenges of caregiving with long-term care options and end-of-life planning to be prepared for the future.

6. And prioritize self-care and build a support network as
   part of your well-being routine.

I invite you to embark on this journey with me, where understanding, compassion, and joy await in the pages of "Dementia
Support for Caregivers and Families." Together, let's make a difference in the lives of those affected by dementia.

1

Unraveling the Mystery: An In-depth Look at Dementia

Lost in the Shadows: The Emotional Journey Through a Loved One's Dementia

In our opening chapter, we delve into the heart-wrenching journey of a daughter grappling with her mother's dementia. Picture her standing in her mother's kitchen, a room once filled with warmth and laughter, now a stage for confusion and misplaced accusations. As she watches her mother, once the pillar of strength and clarity, succumb to the fog of dementia; her heart breaks a little more each day. Her mother, who always remembered the minor details of her daughter's life, now struggles to place her face, mistaking her for a stranger or an unwelcome guest. The daughter's world is turned upside down as she tries to reconcile with this new version of her mother, who remembers her past but not her present (Amy, 2010).

There is another story of Sarah, a beautiful girl who navigates her father's journey through vascular dementia. She noticed subtle changes at first: missed appointments, forgotten birthdays, and confusion over familiar tasks. However, the diagnosis hit her like a wave, leaving her struggling to understand the implications. Vascular dementia, different in its progression from Alzheimer's, presented unique challenges. Sarah had to learn quickly about managing medications, adapting the home environment, and communicating effectively with her father, whose personality changed drastically. Her journey, full of trials, errors, and small victories, highlights the importance of understanding the specific type of dementia your loved one faces.

Like Amy and Sarah, do you find yourself struggling to hold back tears when you see the changes in your loved one's behavior due to dementia? Watching someone who raised you, who was once your advisor and confidante, slip away into a world where you no longer connect can be overwhelmingly painful. How do you cope with the grief and the sense of loss while they are still here, yet so far away?

Embracing the Journey: Understanding and Navigating the Complexities

In this chapter, we address these heartbreaking questions and more. We explore the emotional rollercoaster that family members experience, the practical challenges of caregiving, and the complicated maze of medical and support systems surrounding dementia. Our goal is to offer not just information but also soothing comfort and guidance during what may be one of the most challenging periods of your life.

Dementia is not a singular condition; it's an umbrella term covering conditions of memory decline and loss of communication skills that affect the ability to perform daily activities. Recognizing this diversity is vital to understanding each individual and their family's unique challenges.

In this chapter, we focus on guiding you through both the medical and emotional aspects of dementia. By delving into the various types of dementia, we will provide a comprehensive understanding of the C.A.R.E.S.S. Method. This approach is about grasping the medical facts and empathizing with families' emotional journey. Understanding these complexities is a crucial first step, equipping you with the knowledge and empathy needed to navigate the challenges of dementia care effectively.

Behind the Scenes: The Biological and Neurological Underpinnings of Dementia

What Is Dementia?

Dementia is a term used to describe severe difficulties with memory, language, problem-solving, and other mental abilities. These troubles are severe enough to interrupt living. Most dementia cases are caused by Alzheimer's. However, dementia is a set of symptoms from several illnesses, including Alzheimer's. Due to abnormal brain alterations, cognitive capacities deteriorate, affecting everyday life and independence. Emotions, conduct, and relationships may be affected by dementia (What Is Dementia?, 2019).

Types of Dementia: Exploring the Variants and Their Impact

Dementia is widely recognized for its impact on memory and cognitive function. Understanding the different types of dementia can be crucial for early detection, management, and care. Alzheimer's disease is a widespread kind of dementia, and others include vascular dementia, Lewy body dementia, and frontotemporal dementia. Various illnesses and situations cause other less common varieties of dementia (Types of Dementia, 2023). Let's go into specifics and go over each kind one by one.

1. Alzheimer's Disease

Alzheimer's disease is the most common type of dementia, accounting for an estimated 60-80% of cases. In Alzheimer's disease, the death of brain cells is marked by the presence of amyloid plaques and tau tangles (specific proteins) in the brain. Memory loss in Alzheimer's often starts with recent events before progressing to older memories. Other signs include:

- Difficulty completing familiar tasks.
- Confusion with time or place.
- Trouble with visual images and spatial relationships.

2. Vascular Dementia

Vascular dementia occurs due to blood vessel blockage or damage leading to strokes or bleeding in the brain. The symptoms can be sudden, following a stroke, or gradual, resulting in multiple small strokes. Key indicators include:

- Impaired ability to make decisions.
- Stepwise decline in cognitive abilities.
- Physical symptoms, such as weakness or paralysis.

3. Lewy Body Dementia

Lewy body dementia is characterized by the buildup of Lewy bodies (protein deposits) in nerve cells that affect chemicals in the brain. This can lead to problems with cognition, mobility, behavior, and mood. It is particularly noted for:

- Visual hallucinations.
- Sleep disturbances.
- Parkinsonian movement features.

4. Frontotemporal Dementia

Frontotemporal dementia (FTD) describes disorders caused by nerve cell loss in the brain's frontal or temporal lobes. This type of dementia includes different variants, such as behavioral variant FTD, primary progressive aphasia, and movement disorders. Symptoms vary but can include:

- Changes in personality and behavior.
- Loss of empathy.
- Speech and language difficulties.

5. Mixed Dementia

Mixed dementia occurs when a person has more than one type of dementia. The most common combination is Alzheimer's disease and vascular dementia.

The Fine Line: Separating Typical Aging from Alzheimer's Disease

Alzheimer's disease is a progressive neurological disorder that establishes itself as more than just forgetfulness. Declines in memory and cognition may be severe enough to disrupt daily life, including trouble with familiar tasks, confusion with time or place, and significant challenges in planning or solving problems. Unlike typical memory lapses, Alzheimer's can lead to a person forgetting important dates or information, repeatedly asking the same questions, and experiencing profound mood and personality changes.

On the other hand, typical age-related changes are milder and do not drastically interfere with a person's lifestyle. It is common for elderly individuals to occasionally forget names or appointments, take longer to recall information or make occasional financial errors. Age-related changes can also include temporarily misplacing items but then recalling where to find them, facing challenges when multitasking, or experiencing a slow decline in the ability to process information quickly.

Navigating Dementia with Understanding and Empathy

Knowing how the brain functions and adapts can significantly enhance life for you and your loved ones facing dementia. It's like having a guidebook in a challenging game, making every move more thoughtful and informed. For instance, navigating a new city without a map or GPS can be confusing and stressful. However, with clear directions and a detailed map, the journey becomes more accessible and confident. That is the advantage of understanding dementia. It's like having a navigational tool that helps you manage through its complexities with less anxiety and more clarity.

Understanding the Brain's Structure

The human brain, a remarkable and complex organ, organizes everything we do, from essential functions like breathing to more intricate activities such as moving and thinking. It's where our memories are stored, enabling us to speak and influencing our behavior. The brain's billions of nerve cells are divided into different areas. The largest, the cerebral cortex, is split into other regions, each with its role: the frontal lobes for decision-making and planning, the parietal lobes for processing sensations like touch and spatial awareness, the temporal lobes for handling memory and hearing, and the occipital lobes for vision.

Deep within the brain lies the limbic system, which is vital for our memories and emotions. The cerebellum at the back is key for coordinating movement and balance, while the brainstem at the base controls essential life-sustaining functions such as heartbeat and breathing.

Structural Changes in the Brain due to Dementia

As we have discussed, various areas of the brain are responsible for different cognitive abilities, and when these areas are affected, it leads to the symptoms of dementia. For example, Alzheimer's disease is associated with the buildup of abnormal proteins (plaques and tangles) in the brain, leading to the death of brain cells.

As dementia progresses, it can impact more brain areas, leading to broader changes in personality and behavior. Understanding the connection between the brain and dementia is vital for providing appropriate care for those affected.

Functional Changes in the Brain due to Dementia

In a normal brain, different areas work together smoothly to manage various functions. However, in a brain with dementia, these functions are disrupted, making everyday tasks more challenging. Let's discuss them one by one:

1. **Memory**: The brain can easily recall past events and information. Dementia disrupts this ability, making remembering recent events or learning new information perplexing.

2. **Executive Function** includes planning, organizing, and multitasking skills. A healthy brain manages these tasks efficiently. In dementia, these skills deteriorate, leading to difficulties in managing daily activities and making decisions.

3. **Vision**: The brain usually interprets what we see accurately. Dementia can alter this, causing problems with depth perception, distinguishing colors, or recognizing familiar faces and objects. Vision also gets tricky. The brain does more than see; it interprets what we see by connecting it to memories. So, someone with dementia might have healthy eyes but still have trouble recognizing faces or objects.

4. **Language**: In a normal brain, finding the right words and understanding others is effortless. Dementia affects these abilities, making it hard to communicate effectively, both in speaking and understanding.

5. **Emotion**: Typically, the brain regulates emotions appropriately. However, with dementia, unexpected emotional responses or mood swings might occur, making it difficult to control feelings.

6. **Behavior**: A healthy brain helps maintain consistent and socially appropriate behavior. Dementia can change how people feel and behave. The parts of the brain that handle emotions and rational thinking can get mixed up, leading to unexpected reactions like laughing at sad news or feeling anxious for no apparent reason.

Stages of Dementia

Dementia, a progressive condition characterized by declining cognitive function, manifests differently across its stages and varies between individuals. Understanding the different stages of dementia is vital for providing personalized and effective care, as it helps caregivers and healthcare providers tailor their support to the specific needs and abilities of the individual at each stage. Let's delve into different stages of dementia:

Early Stage of Dementia

In the early stage, symptoms are often mild, affecting specific abilities depending on the part of the brain initially impacted (10 Early Signs and Symptoms of Alzheimer's and Dementia, 2024). Common symptoms include:

- **Memory Loss:** Memory loss, particularly of recent events, is a characteristic symptom of dementia. It starts with seemingly minor forgetfulness, like misplacing items or forgetting names and appointments, but unlike typical age-related memory lapses, these are not usually remembered later. For instance, a person with dementia may repeatedly forget recent conversations or appointments and not recall them at all, even after a short period.
- **Impaired ability to focus, pay attention, plan, and organize:** This impairment often manifests in everyday activities, like managing finances or household bills. For example, a person with dementia may struggle with planning a budget, forget to pay bills, or make calculation errors, which differs from the occasional mistakes seen in normal aging.
- **Difficulty with communication and language:** This is a common early symptom of dementia, progressing from mild to more severe forms. Initially, it may involve challenges like finding the right word during conversations. As dementia advances, these difficulties

increase. Individuals may frequently substitute incorrect words, making their speech hard to understand. They might quickly lose their train of thought, making conversing difficult.

- **Confusion and Misunderstanding:** In dementia, misunderstanding what is seen and confusion about time or place are notable symptoms. Individuals may have trouble recognizing familiar faces or objects, or they might misinterpret visual information, leading to challenges in navigating even well-known environments. Confusion about time or place is also prevalent. For instance, a person with dementia might frequently become unsure about the day of the week.

- **Poor Judgment and Mood Swings:** Poor judgment leading to bad decisions is a common symptom in the progression of dementia. This could manifest as neglecting personal hygiene, making unwise financial decisions, or a departure from the person's previous decision-making abilities. Additionally, changes in mood and personality are frequently observed.

- **Difficult recognition of objects and people:** Difficulty recognizing objects and people indicates a cognitive decline associated with dementia. This difficulty can lead to misplacing everyday items, a symptom that goes beyond the typical forgetfulness of occasionally losing keys or a wallet. For instance, a person with dementia might frequently put things in unusual places and then be unable to retrace their steps to find them.

- **Challenges in Planning or Problem-Solving:** This symptom affects the ability to develop and execute plans, like organizing a schedule or managing finances. Tasks requiring multiple steps or concentration, such as following recipes or tracking monthly bills, become challenging.

Middle Stage of Dementia

The middle stage of dementia can be the most extended phase and presents more noticeable and challenging symptoms (The Middle Stage of Dementia, 2021):

- **Aggressive Behavior:** As dementia progresses, individuals may exhibit aggression, which can be verbal (shouting, using harsh words) or physical (hitting, pushing). For example, a person might become aggressive when feeling overwhelmed or misunderstood during daily care routines, such as bathing.
- **Wandering:** People in the middle stages of dementia might walk aimlessly within the home or leave the house at odd hours. An example is a person with dementia repeatedly pacing the hallway at night or wandering outside, searching for a 'safe' place or a long-gone childhood home.
- **Lack of Insight:** This refers to the reduced awareness of their cognitive decline. For instance, someone with dementia might insist on driving, unaware of their impaired abilities, or deny needing any help despite clear signs of struggling with daily tasks.
- **Sleep Problems:** Disturbed sleep patterns become more common. An individual with dementia might wake up frequently during the night or start wandering around the house, mistaking night for day.
- **Delusions:** Delusional thinking can lead to false beliefs. For example, a person might accuse family members of stealing items they have misplaced or believe a spouse is unfaithful without any evidence.

- **Increased Memory Loss and Confusion:** Memory issues become more prominent, with significant difficulty recalling personal history, recent events, or recognizing friends and family. Confusion about time and place becomes more frequent.
- **Impaired Judgment and Decision Making:** People may show poor judgment in personal care or financial decisions and struggle with complex tasks.
- **Challenges with Daily Activities:** Increased dependence on others for personal care tasks, such as dressing, bathing, and toileting. There might be a decreased appetite or difficulty in eating.

During the middle stage, support from caregivers becomes increasingly crucial as individuals lose the ability to perform daily tasks independently. Understanding and patience are vital to managing these challenges effectively.

Late Stage of Dementia

In the later stages of dementia, the condition significantly impacts a person's life, requiring full-time care and support, especially with daily living activities (The Later Stage of Dementia, 2021). Symptoms become more severe, extensively affecting a person's everyday life. This stage is characterized by:

- **Profound Memory Loss:** Individuals may lose the ability to recognize family and friends and often seem to be living in a different time period. Their long-term memory might also fade, affecting even deeply ingrained memories.
- **Severe Communication Difficulties:** The ability to speak diminishes significantly. They might rely on non-verbal communication, like facial expressions or gestures.

Understanding what others say can also become extremely difficult.

- **Physical Decline:** Mobility decreases, often leading to wheelchair use or bed-bound states. Eating and swallowing difficulties are common, increasing the risk of choking or developing pneumonia. Assistance with all physical activities becomes necessary.
- **Walk More Slowly:** Some people walk with a shuffle, moving more slowly and unsteadily. This often leads to increased time spent in a chair or bed.
- **Increased Risk of Falling:** Due to decreased mobility and balance, there is a heightened risk of falls, which can lead to severe injuries.
- **Needing Help with Eating:** As dementia progresses, people may need substantial assistance with eating, often resulting in weight loss due to eating difficulties.
- **Difficulty in Swallowing:** Swallowing problems can arise, increasing the risk of choking or aspiration pneumonia.
- **Total Dependence on Care:** Complete reliance on caregivers for personal care, including feeding, bathing, and toileting. Care at this stage focuses on maintaining comfort, dignity, and quality of life.

In the late stage, care focuses on comfort, pain management, and maintaining the individual's dignity.

Variability in Dementia Progression

The progression of dementia varies significantly from person to person, influenced by factors such as the type of dementia, individual brain differences, age, overall health, and other medical conditions. For example, Alzheimer's disease typically progresses more slowly than other forms of dementia, and its rate of progression can differ based on age and the presence of other health issues. Furthermore, the specific area of the brain initially affected by dementia determines the early symptoms and their severity, contributing to the variability in progression among individuals (The Progression, Signs and Stages of Dementia, 2021).

Unveiling the Roots: Investigating the Causes and Prevention Strategies for Dementia

Causes of Dementia

Dementia is caused by the brain's loss of nerve cell connections, which various factors can trigger. Each type of dementia may have different underlying causes:

- **Alzheimer's Disease:** The most common cause of dementia, Alzheimer's is marked by an accumulation of plaques and tangles in the brain. These formations damage healthy brain cells and their connections. Genetic factors, such as mutations in specific genes, contribute to the risk of developing Alzheimer's (Dementia - Symptoms and Causes, 2023).
- **Vascular Dementia:** This type occurs due to damage of blood vessels that supply the brain. Conditions like stroke or atherosclerosis (buildup of fats in artery walls) can reduce blood flow to the brain, leading to symptoms like problem-solving difficulties, slowed thinking, and memory issues.
- **Lewy Body Dementia:** Characterized by the presence of Lewy bodies, which are balloon-like clumps of protein found in the brain. Symptoms include visual hallucinations, movement disorders, and cognitive issues.

- **Frontotemporal Dementia:** Involves the breakdown of nerve cells in the frontal and temporal lobes of the brain, affecting areas responsible for personality, behavior, and language. This leads to changes in behavior, personality, and language skills.
- **Huntington's Disease:** A genetic disorder that negatively affects nerve cells in the brain and spinal cord, leading to cognitive decline, movement control issues, and personality changes (Clinic, 2022).
- **Traumatic Brain Injury:** Repeated head trauma, such as that experienced by athletes or in accidents, can lead to dementia. Symptoms may include memory decline, mood changes, and speech difficulties.
- **Creutzfeldt-Jakob Disease:** This rare condition is caused by prions, infectious proteins that lead to the death of nerve cells in the brain. Symptoms include cognitive and behavioral changes, confusion, and depression.
- **Parkinson's Disease Dementia:** Develops in the later stages of Parkinson's disease, affecting memory and thinking abilities along with typical Parkinson's symptoms like tremors and slow movement.
- **Wernicke-Korsakoff Syndrome:** Caused by a severe deficiency of thiamine (vitamin B1), often related to alcohol use disorder. It can result in bleeding in brain areas critical for memory.
- **Infections and Immune Disorders:** Some infections and immune system disorders can cause dementia-like symptoms. This includes conditions like multiple sclerosis and diseases such as late-stage syphilis.
- **Normal-Pressure Hydrocephalus:** This condition is caused by the buildup of cerebrospinal fluid in the brain's ventricles. It leads to memory loss, incontinence and

mobility problems, memory loss, and loss of bladder control.

Risk Factors of Dementia

The risk factors for dementia can be categorized into those that cannot be changed and those that lifestyle choices and health management can influence. Let's discuss each of them:

- **Age:** Age is the most significant risk factor for dementia. The likelihood of developing dementia increases with age, particularly after 65 years. While dementia is more common in older age, it is not a normal part of aging, and younger individuals can be affected as well.
- **Genetics:** Having a family history of dementia increases the risk. Specific genetic mutations, such as those related to Alzheimer's disease, can be inherited. However, not everyone with a family history of dementia will develop it, and many without a family history do as well.
- **Lifestyle Choices:** Lifestyle factors, such as smoking, significantly affect the risk of developing dementia. Smoking can increase the risk of dementia and vascular diseases, which in turn impact brain health. Additionally, excessive alcohol consumption and a sedentary lifestyle are also risk factors.
- **Diabetes:** People with diabetes, mainly if poorly controlled, have an increased risk of dementia. Diabetes can lead to vascular complications, which affect blood flow to the brain and may impact the development of vascular dementia.

Lifestyle changes and regular interactions with your physician can help reduce the risk of developing dementia. For instance, quitting smoking, maintaining a healthy diet, regular exercise, and effective management of diabetes can contribute to better brain health and lower the risk of dementia.

Preventing Dementia

Preventing dementia, especially for those not genetically predisposed, involves a multifaceted approach focusing on various aspects of lifestyle and health management. Here are detailed strategies suggested by (Robinson, 2018):

- **Regular Exercise:** Physical activity is crucial in reducing the risk of Alzheimer's and other types of dementia. Regular exercise of at least 20-30 minutes daily of moderate-intensity exercise, including cardio and strength training, helps maintain brain health. Activities suitable for beginners, like walking and swimming, are also suitable.
- **Social Engagement:** Maintaining strong social connections is vital for brain health. Regular, meaningful face-to-face interactions can protect against Alzheimer's and dementia symptoms. Volunteering, joining clubs, attending community or senior centers, and staying connected with friends and neighbors are recommended.
- **Healthy Diet:** To reduce the risk of cognitive decline, try to consume a diet low in sugar and rich in fruits, vegetables, whole grains, and omega-3 fatty acids. The Mediterranean diet is associated with a reduced risk of Alzheimer's and dementia. This diet emphasizes vegetables, beans, whole grains, fish, and olive oil and limits processed foods. Managing weight and reducing intake of sugary and refined carbs are also important.
- **Mental Stimulation:** Continuously challenging the brain through learning and cognitive engagement is crucial. This

includes learning new skills, engaging in complex tasks that require communication and organization, and enjoying brain-stimulating activities like puzzles and strategy games.

- **Quality Sleep:** Good sleep is essential for brain health. Poor sleep as a habit has been linked to higher levels of amyloid (a protein associated with Alzheimer's). Creating a relaxing bedtime routine, making a sleep schedule, and addressing sleep disorders like sleep apnea can improve sleep quality, supporting cognitive health.
- **Stress Management:** Stress can negatively impact the brain, increasing the risk of Alzheimer's and dementia. Yoga, meditation, and breathing exercises are excellent stress management techniques. Engaging in enjoyable activities, especially with family and friends, can help ease the effects of stress on the brain. Maintaining a sense of humor and prioritizing fun activities are also beneficial.
- **Vascular Health:** Good cardiovascular health is closely linked to brain health. Controlling blood pressure and cholesterol levels, avoiding smoking, and following a heart-healthy diet can reduce dementia risk. High blood pressure and high cholesterol are associated with an increased risk of dementia.

These strategies encompass a holistic approach to health and well-being, emphasizing the importance of a balanced lifestyle for reducing the risk of dementia. It's essential to consult healthcare providers for personalized advice and to manage any existing health conditions effectively.

Treatment of Dementia

Treating dementia involves a multi-pronged approach to managing symptoms while maintaining quality of life, as there is currently no cure for most types of dementia. The treatment strategies include:

- **Medications:** Cholinesterase inhibitors, such as donepezil, rivastigmine, and galantamine, boost chemical messengers involved in memory and judgment. They are primarily used in Alzheimer's disease but may also be prescribed for other types of dementia. Side effects include gastrointestinal issues, slowed heart rate, and sleep problems. Memantine is used to regulate the activity of glutamate chemical messenger involved in learning and memory. Lecanemab is the new drug approved by the FDA in 2023 for mild Alzheimer's disease and mild cognitive impairment (Dementia - Diagnosis and Treatment - Mayo Clinic, 2023).
- **Therapies:** Occupational therapy helps make the home environment safer and teaches coping behaviors to prevent accidents and manage behavior changes. Simplifying tasks and reducing clutter and noise can also help individuals with dementia to focus and function better. Therapies like music therapy, pet therapy, aromatherapy, and art therapy can be helpful; however, the effectiveness of dietary supplements and herbal remedies is not conclusively proven, and caution is advised, especially if other medications are being taken.
- **Communication and Exercise:** Using simple sentences, maintaining eye contact, and giving time to respond can improve interaction. Physical activities can improve

strength, balance, and cardiovascular health. It may also help with restlessness and depression.

It's important to note that the medications used in dementia treatment primarily aim to slow down the progression of symptoms rather than cure the disease. Each patient's experience with dementia is unique. So, each person's treatment plan and care plan should be tailored to individual needs, considering the stage of dementia, other health conditions, and personal preferences.

Busting the Myths: Dispelling Common Misconceptions Surrounding Dementia

Here are the common misconceptions about dementia, addressed with factual, research-supported information:

1. Misconception: Dementia is a disease.

Reality: Dementia is not a disease but instead describes a group of symptoms affecting the ability to think, remember, and reason to a degree that impairs daily living activities. It also includes changes in language, communication, mood, and behavior (5 Myths about Dementia | Pfizer, 2023).

2. Misconception: Memory loss is the first sign of dementia.

Reality: While dementia does involve memory issues affecting daily functioning, memory loss is not necessarily the first symptom. Unexplained mood, behavior, or ability changes can also be early signs and warrant a doctor visit (5 Common Misconceptions about Dementia | Alzheimer's Foundation of America, 2021).

3. Misconception: Dementia is a natural part of aging.

Reality: While dementia is expected in the aging population, it is not a standard or natural part of aging. Aging might bring reduced physical and mental agility, but dementia is a distinct medical condition (5 Common Misconceptions about Dementia | Alzheimer's Foundation of America, 2021).

4. Misconception: Dementia is always genetic.

Reality: Some forms of dementia, like early-onset Alzheimer's, have a stronger genetic link due to inherited gene mutations. However, most dementia cases result from a combination of genetics, lifestyle, and environmental factors. Genetics are a variable risk factor depending on the type and cause of dementia (Is Dementia Hereditary? 2023).

5. Misconception: Dementia causes the loss of all memories.

Reality: Dementia's impact on memory can vary widely among individuals. While some may lose many memories, others may retain significant aspects of their past experiences.

6. Misconception: Dementia-like symptoms are never reversible.

Reality: Some brain disorders causing cognitive impairment or dementia-like symptoms can be reversed if the primary cause is addressed. These include conditions related to toxic, autoimmune, infectious, metabolic, and vitamin deficiencies, certain medical conditions like chronic subdural hematomas, alcohol use disorder, early-treated Lyme disease, untreated sleep apnea, and psychiatric disorders (Nathan. K, 2022).

7. Misconception: All types of dementia are the same.

Reality: There are many different types of dementia, such as Alzheimer's dementia, Parkinson's dementia, vascular dementia, Lewy Body dementia, and frontotemporal dementia, each with unique characteristics and symptoms (5 Myths about Dementia | Pfizer, 2023).

8. Misconception: Dementia is usually diagnosed shortly after the onset of Alzheimer's disease.

Reality: Dementia-causing diseases can be present up to 20 years before dementia symptoms begin. Early signs are often mild cognitive impairments that might not cause concern initially (5 Myths about Dementia | Pfizer, 2023).

9. Misconception: You can tell someone has dementia because they cannot communicate and usually live in a facility.

Reality: The progression of dementia, especially due to Alzheimer's, is gradual. Many people with dementia live independently with moderate help and manage their lives effectively (5 Myths about Dementia | Pfizer, 2023).

10. Misconception: Only older people get dementia.

Reality: While more common in older individuals, dementia can also affect younger people. Young-onset Alzheimer's and frontotemporal dementia can affect people as young as in their 50s or earlier (5 Common Misconceptions about Dementia | Alzheimer's Foundation of America, 2021).

11. Misconception: People with dementia become agitated, violent, and aggressive.

Reality: Not all individuals with dementia exhibit agitation, violence, or aggression. Dementia affects each person differently, and such behaviors often result from confusion, fear, or unmet needs (5 Common Misconceptions about Dementia | Alzheimer's Foundation of America, 2021).

12. Misconception: People with dementia can't enjoy new activities, learn new things, or have a good quality of life.

Reality: Many people with dementia continue to have meaningful lives, enjoying activities, learning new routines, and experiencing love and joy. The key is adapting activities and relying on support from others (5 Common Misconceptions about Dementia | Alzheimer's Foundation of America, 2021).

13. Misconception: Nothing can be done for dementia.

Reality: Early diagnosis of dementia allows for treatments and therapies that may slow progression. Focusing on abilities and joy rather than declines and losses is crucial (5 Common Misconceptions about Dementia | Alzheimer's Foundation of America, 2021).

We have navigated the complex and emotional landscape of dementia through the intricacies of its various forms, the challenges it poses to individuals and their families, and the scientific underpinning that defines its progression. This exploration has offered a deeper understanding of dementia and a testament to the resilience and courage of those who live in its shadow.

Transitioning from the shadows of dementia, we pivot to a brighter chapter, adaptation through mastering communication. If understanding dementia is like mapping the terrain of an unknown territory, mastering communication is the art of navigating this terrain with grace and effectiveness. In the upcoming chapter, we will explore the transformative power of communication in caregiving and beyond. We will delve into how effective communication strategies can bridge the gap between confusion and clarity, foster deep connections, and provide solace and understanding amid dementia's challenges.

Mastering communication encompasses non-verbal cues, emotional intelligence, and the ability to listen with empathy. It's about finding new ways to connect when traditional paths are obscured, creating moments of joy and recognition in a landscape marked by confusion.

As we transition to this new chapter, we carry forward the insights gained from our deep dive into dementia, ready to apply them in the quest to enhance our interactions and relationships with those we care for. Through mastering communication, we will light a beacon of hope, illuminating the path forward for both caregivers and those embarking on the dementia journey.

2

The Art of Adaptation

Mastering Communication

I magine yourself standing at the crossroads of compassion and understanding, where each word you speak and every action you take becomes a powerful tool in bridging the ever-widening gap created by dementia. This chapter is not just about learning techniques; it is about transforming your approach to care. As dementia reshapes the landscape of your loved one's reality, your ability to adapt your communication and behavior management strategies becomes an example of illumination in their world of growing shadows. Together, we will explore practical, heart-centered skills grounded in the latest research and enriched by real-life experiences. These skills will improve your effectiveness as a caregiver. They will also deepen the emotional connection with your loved one, making every moment count in this journey of love, challenge, and profound learning.

Dementia profoundly impacts communication, altering the ability to speak, write, understand, and interpret language. As dementia progresses, individuals may create new words for forgotten ones, get stuck on a word or phrase, or struggle to find the right word. They may face difficulties in reading and writing or revert to their first language. They commonly lose their train of thought and have trouble expressing themselves and understanding spoken words. Following complex instructions or staying on topic may become challenging, even impossible.

Moreover, dementia can also cause sensory changes, such as hypersensitivity to noise and certain tones, further complicating communication with environmental factors. These changes can be upsetting and frustrating, not just for the person with dementia but also for their caregivers, friends, and family (Communication Challenges and Helpful Strategies, 2022).

Finding Unspoken Words: Emma's Journey with Dementia Care.

In this context, imagine Emma, who cares for her mother with advanced dementia. Each day brings new challenges as her mother's ability to communicate diminishes. Emma notices that her mother often repeats phrases, struggles to find the right words, and sometimes reverts to her native language, which Emma does not fully understand. During their conversations, her mother frequently loses her train of thought and becomes visibly frustrated and anxious when she cannot express herself clearly. These communication barriers leave Emma feeling helpless and emotionally drained as she struggles to understand her mother's needs and emotions.

Emma has found that specific strategies can improve communication. For instance, she encourages her mother to express her wishes and plans, which gives her a sense of control and eases the family's concerns. In social situations, Emma gently prompts her mother to stay on topic, asks people to speak slowly and clearly, and uses simple, short sentences to avoid overwhelming her. Recognizing the increasing importance of non-verbal communication, Emma uses visual aids, gestures, and body language to enhance their interaction. She also uses a tablet to help her mother record her thoughts and write letters, which has been particularly effective in helping her communicate more effectively.

Caring for her mother, Emma realizes that dementia's impact on communication is profound, requiring patience, understanding, and adaptability. Through these challenges, she remains committed to supporting her mother in living as fulfilling a life as possible despite the barriers imposed by dementia.

Joel's Journey: Embracing the Echoes of Memory

In a small town with hills and woods, there lived a man named Joel. He had countless stories from his past, many about the town's history. However, Joel started to forget some of those stories as he got older. It was like his memory was fading away. His dementia journey was confusing and uncertain.

At first, he forgot names and where he put things like his keys. But as time passed, it became even more challenging for him to remember things. His family, including his wife Sarah, son Michael, and granddaughter Lily, had to deal with this new situation. They watched as Joel, who used to guide them through life, started to act like a child. Sarah was like a guiding light for him, helping him through the confusion with her love. Michael was sad to see his dad change but tried to accept the new Joel. Lily found a special connection with her grandpa. She saw his forgetfulness as a way for him to use his imagination freely (Three real life stories of dementia, 2021). Altering beliefs about how Dad or Grandpa should be, based on how he used to be, gives both the caregiver and the person with dementia the space to grow and change with dignity. Lily's ability to see her grandpa's dementia as a new freedom for imagination creates an environment of discovery and joy.

This chapter focuses on Step 2, emphasizing the 'A' in C.A.R.E.S.S., which stands for Adaptation through understanding and interpreting dementia communication. With techniques to help you effectively interact with a person with dementia, this begins your adaptation and personal growth journey. It is about learning these virtues in theory and integrating them into the fabric of your caregiving practice, transforming challenges into opportunities for deeper connection and personal growth.

Navigating the Maze: Decoding the Language of Dementia

The language changes in individuals with dementia can be affected by many factors, including the personality of individuals, the type of dementia they have, and the stage of the disease. Let us see how language changes in individuals with dementia based on different factors:

1. Individual's Personality

A person's personality and how they manage these language problems also play a significant role. For instance, some individuals might become more withdrawn or frustrated due to difficulty expressing themselves or understanding others. Additionally, they may experience a deterioration in their reading and writing skills and have difficulty adhering to the usual social conventions of conversation, such as increasing tendencies to interrupt or ignore a speaker (Dementia - Communication, 2014).

Caregivers are encouraged to connect with the person, foster independence, and assist as needed. This approach helps maintain the individual's engagement and can create positive emotions, reducing anxiety and fear (Understanding the Barriers, 2018).

2. Type of Dementia

The specific type of dementia greatly influences language problems. For instance, in some forms of frontotemporal dementia (FTD), language issues can appear much earlier than in other types of dementia and may be one of the first symptoms noticed.

3. Stage of Dementia

The stage of dementia also plays a crucial role. As dementia progresses, the individual's ability to communicate and use language effectively can deteriorate significantly. This deterioration can impact their ability to respond appropriately or follow a conversation. Due to difficulties in understanding, focusing, and thinking speed, constructing a reply will become more difficult for the sufferer. It is essential to consider that dementia can lead to behaviors like making inappropriate comments, repeating questions, or holding false beliefs, which are all part of communication challenges (Dementia & Language, 2023).

4. External Factors

External factors like physical health, pain, discomfort, or medication side effects can affect communication. For example, a sudden behavior change, like a marked increase in confusion, could indicate a medical emergency, such as an infection or injury. Too much visual stimulation and too many choices can cause confusion, so re-organize the environment and put away unused and unnecessary items to create a more peaceful environment.

Communication Barriers in Dementia

Barriers in dementia care can significantly impact the communication between family members and their loved ones with dementia. Based on the information from the Wesbury Retirement Community website, these barriers can be categorized as follows (Understanding the Barriers, 2018):

1. Caregiver's Communication Style:

The person with dementia requires a specific approach. Caregivers should approach from the front, introduce themselves, speak slowly, and be patient. Using simple language and being mindful of body language is crucial. It is essential not to make assumptions about the person's abilities and to speak directly to them. Making eye contact at their level and minimizing distractions can facilitate better communication.

2. Physical Environment:

The environment plays a significant role in communication for someone with dementia. A well-planned environment that limits noise and distractions can help the person focus. This involves improving lighting, reducing unsettling sounds and crowds, and fostering independence by minimizing clutter and ensuring clear paths to frequently used areas like the bathroom.

3. Lack of Activity and Purposeful Engagement:

Engaging the person with dementia in activities can be a good form of communication. Every task or interaction should be viewed as an opportunity for activity, giving them a sense of purpose. This maintains their skills and abilities, reduces challenging behaviors, and can improve sleep.

4. Not Recognizing Their Behaviour as Communication:

It is essential to understand that behaviors exhibited by a person with dementia are often purposeful and a form of communication. Caregivers need to look for the meaning behind behaviors and consider factors like discomfort due to temperature, hunger, thirst, pain, toileting issues, or boredom. Recognizing these behaviors as a form of communication can lead to better understanding and care.

5. Caregiver Approach:

The approach taken by the caregiver is fundamental. The focus should be connecting with the loved one first, not just accomplishing a task. Encouraging independence and assisting only when necessary is important to maintaining dignity. When caregivers interact with the person with dementia, it helps the individual stay active and engaged, prevents anxiety or fear, enhances enjoyment, and fosters positive emotions.

14 Strategies to Communicate Effectively with a Person with Dementia

Communicating effectively with dementia involves several strategies that can significantly improve the interaction and overall well-being of the person with dementia and the caregiver. Here are the strategies, and let's discuss them in detail (How to Communicate with a Person with Dementia, 2021).

1. Setting a Positive Environment for Interaction

Creating a comfortable and positive environment is crucial when interacting with someone with dementia. Approach them with a smile and maintain a pleasant, affectionate tone. This helps create a relaxed atmosphere and makes communication easier. For instance, when sitting down to chat, ensure the lighting is gentle and the seating is comfortable. Speak soothingly, using phrases filled with warmth and affection. This approach makes them feel at ease and opens avenues for smoother communication.

2. Getting the Person's Attention

Minimizing distractions is a key to effective communication. Before starting a conversation, ensure the environment is conducive to focused interaction. This could mean turning off the TV or closing the door to a noisy room. Approach the person calmly, address them by name, and introduce yourself each time to avoid confusion. For example, saying "Hi Dad, it's Anna" helps orient them to who you are and your relationship with them, making them more receptive to the conversation.

3. Listening Carefully

Listening is as essential as speaking. Pay close attention to what the person with dementia tries to express verbally and non-verbally. This involves acknowledging their feelings and responding with empathy. Showing that you actively listen through nods and verbal affirmations encourages them to share more and feel heard.

4. Communicating Clearly

When talking to a person with dementia, speaking clearly and using straightforward language is essential. Avoid using complex sentences or jargon that may need to be clarified. Keep your tone friendly and use familiar words. For instance, instead of saying, "Are you thinking about having something to eat?" you can ask, "Are you hungry?"

5. Using Short, Simple Sentences

Simplicity is vital in communication. Use short, simple sentences to convey your messages. This makes it easier for the person with dementia to follow along and understand. For instance, instead of saying, "Would you prefer to have the chicken soup or the vegetable stew for your meal?" ask, "Do you want chicken soup?"

6. Being Patient and Respectful

Patience and respect are fundamental. Understand that communication might take more time and effort. Give them time to process and respond and avoid interrupting or finishing their sentences. This shows respect for their efforts and encourages more interaction.

7. Being Mindful of Your Tone

A calm, soothing, and lower-pitched voice can be comforting and easier to understand. This is particularly important when the person is anxious or confused.

8. Communicating at a Slower Pace

Speak slowly and distinctly. This gives the person more time to process the words and reduces the likelihood of misunderstanding. Pausing between sentences also helps them catch up and keeps them engaged in the conversation.

9. Allowing the Person to Complete Their Sentences

Encourage them to express themselves fully, even if they take time to complete their sentences. Please resist the urge to speak for them or finish their thoughts. This helps us better understand their needs and promotes their sense of independence and dignity.

10. Using and Understanding Body Language

Non-verbal cues are crucial in communication. Sustain eye contact and use facial demonstrations and gentle physical touches to express your message and affection. For instance, a reassuring touch on the arm or a warm smile can significantly aid communication. If the person is seated, stoop or sit down to their level to make eye contact and interaction more personal and respectful.

11. Avoiding Complicated Questions

Ask simple, direct questions that are easy to understand and respond to. Avoid open-ended questions that might be confusing. Instead of asking, "What would you like to do today?" you can ask more straightforward questions like, "Would you like to go outside for a walk?"

12. Sticking to One Idea at a Time

Discuss one topic at a time to prevent confusion. This helps the person with dementia to stay focused and engaged in the conversation. It is also easier for them to process and respond to one piece of information at a time.

13. Paraphrasing Questions Appropriately

Tailor your questions to the stage of their dementia. In the early stages, open-ended questions encourage more conversation. For example, "What would you like for breakfast?" In the middle stages, offer limited choices to make decision-making more accessible, like "Would you like tea or coffee?" In the late stages, use yes/no questions or provide a guided choice, such as "Do you like this music? Let's keep it playing."

14. Using Communication Therapies

Different communication therapies can be highly effective. Validation therapy involves acknowledging their feelings and experiences, creating a sense of empathy. Music therapy can be soothing and stimulating; engage them in singing familiar songs or listening to music they enjoy.

The 10 Absolutes to Improve Communication

The "10 Absolutes of Alzheimer's Care" by Jo Huey (@Huey, 1996) offers vital principles for communicating with individuals with dementia. Practice of these simple rules will ease daily tasks and create positive interactions, turning struggles into loving interactions. These principles are demonstrated by combining practical strategies with personal stories from caregivers to illustrate their effectiveness.

1. Never Argue, Instead Agree:

Dementia can alter a person's perception of reality. I remember a resident in the early stages of dementia at our nursing home who often experienced sundowning (a common symptom where confusion and anxiety increase in the afternoon hours). While we were setting up for dinner one evening, she entered the dining room, visibly distressed. "I missed the train. What should I do now? How can I catch up and get back on it? Oh, I have really messed things up this time," she lamented, anxiously wringing her hands.

To calm her, we reassured her, "Do not worry, this is an overnight stay. Everyone from the train is having dinner here and has been assigned a room for the night. The train won't return tonight. You are right where you need to be." Although she was initially doubt-ful, showing her the room and accompanying her back to the dining room for dinner helped. Prioritizing her peace of mind over strict truthfulness, we watched as she gradually relaxed, enjoyed her meal, and had a restful night. This approach shows the value of validating the patient's feelings and entering their reality to foster a peaceful environment.

2. Never Reason, Instead Divert:

Reasoning with someone with dementia can be ineffective due to their impaired cognitive abilities. The story of Paul shows the benefit of gently shifting the focus. One Sunday morning, I received an urgent call from a close friend whose husband (Paul) was battling Lewy Body Dementia. She needed help as he was becoming unmanageable. Upon arriving, I found him visibly agitated, seated at the dining table. Recognizing me, he exclaimed, "Thank God you are here. I don't know these clowns," gesturing towards his wife and son. "They keep forcing me to do things. I don't recognize them, and I don't trust them," he said, his voice filled with distress.

To defuse the situation, I casually remarked, "Let's ignore them for now. They seem occupied anyway. How about we have a chat?" I explained that I was nearby and wanted to see how he was doing. This diverted his attention away from his family, whom he perceived as strangers. Noticing his uneaten breakfast and medication on the table, I gently encouraged him, "Don't mind me. Please go ahead with your pills and breakfast." He had previously refused to eat or take medication from his family. He took his pills without further comment and began to enjoy his meal.

Engaging in light conversation for a few minutes, I casually complimented on the appealing look of his breakfast. I reminisced that he often told me he married his wife for her excellent cooking skills. "You chose well; she's a great cook!" I added. This comment triggered a recognition. He looked around, saw his wife in the kitchen, and affectionately said, "Well, there she is."

He was early in his Lewy Body Dementia journey, and everyone is different, but he did not 'forget' his wife again for some time. It is all about acknowledging their feelings and providing a sense of familiarity and safety.

3. Never Shame, Instead Distract:

Shaming can exacerbate anxiety and confusion in dementia patients. The strategy of engaging Sasha illustrates how distraction with familiar and enjoyable activities can be soothing. Sasha tended to pace incessantly, which seemed to heighten her anxiety. To alleviate this, we would join her on her walks, engage her in conversation, and admire her fitness. Compliments had a calming effect on her. Knowing that she used to enjoy walking around her neighborhood, we tried to take her outside whenever possible, offering companionship while ensuring her safety.

Occasionally, we would suggest a break, inviting her to sit and share a soda with us. This simple act of sitting and chatting over a drink often provided a much-needed respite for her. Engaging her in conversations about her past interests proved beneficial, too. For instance, she was an avid gardener. We would talk about the joy of gardening, asking her about her experiences and preferences.

To help her relax further, we employed visualization techniques. We would talk about the feeling of soil in our hands, encouraging her to close her eyes and imagine the sensation and smell of the earth. This method of redirecting her focus from her anxieties to more pleasant, familiar sensations proved to be a soothing and effective strategy.

4. Never Lecture, Instead Reassure:

Lecturing can be overwhelming for someone with dementia. This case highlights the effectiveness of reassurance in alleviating anxiety and fear. One morning, a 90-year-old woman approached me, visibly upset and fearful. Concerned, I asked her about the cause of her distress. She confided, "I am in so much trouble. I've been out all night, and it's already morning. My mother is going to be so unforgiving. I am in deep trouble!" To alleviate her anxiety, I reassured her gently, telling her that her mother was not there and was unaware of the situation. I suggested, "Let's keep this our little secret. Your mom doesn't have to know." This seemed to comfort her, and she could continue her day, feeling more at ease.

In another example, Bruce's father, with dementia, began hiding his dirty underwear in his dresser with clean clothes. At first, Bruce was horrified and upset, but he managed the situation by doing several things. He began checking with his dad several times daily to ask if he needed to go to the bathroom. He 'remodeled' Dad's room, removing the dresser and replacing it with a table and chairs, which they used for puzzle time. He began setting out clothes for the day and leaving only one change in the room. He did not lecture his dad or try to get him to understand; he gave reassurance. Presenting these as positive changes for his dad helped gain his agreement and cooperation.

5. Never Say 'Remember,' Instead Reminisce:

Directly asking dementia patients to recall recent events can frustrate them. This anecdote describes that discussing long-term memories can help build connections and reduce anxiety. A gentleman was new to our nursing home. A new setting is always the most difficult. He was confused, anxious, and angry. Attempting to make a connection, I asked about his wife and children. He just looked at me with a blank stare. So, I then asked how many brothers and sisters he had. He completely relaxed and told me about his family life, going into detail about where and how he grew up. It was fascinating to listen to, and we became 'old friends,' making a lasting connection. This approach fosters a sense of comfort and familiarity, making new environments feel more welcoming.

6. Never Say 'I told you,' Instead Repeat:

Repetition is crucial in communicating with dementia patients. Doing so patiently and without making them feel incompetent respects their dignity and helps them feel understood and supported. Dementia patients cannot help the fact that they do not remember something you may have told them five minutes ago. By accepting that you will need to repeat a thing many times as a fact, you gain access to repeat yourself with patience, compassion, and cheerfulness.

7. Never Say 'You can't,' Instead Say 'Do what you can':

Focusing on a dementia patient's abilities, rather than limitations, empowers them. Let's see an example: Mary, one of our residents, prepared herself one morning for a doctor's appointment with a sense of pride. She chose to wear a revealing summer top, not realizing it was too cold outside and inappropriate attire. Instead of dismissing her choice, we offered a practical yet respectful solution. We suggested adding a sweater over her top, complimenting her on how cute she looked. This approach allowed us to ensure her comfort without undermining her choice, thus preserving her dignity.

In another instance, an 85-year-old resident expressed a unique wish: to get her ears pierced, but not at a mall or doctor's office. She was set on visiting a tattoo shop for this experience. Honoring her preference, we arranged an appointment at a tattoo shop. The experience turned out to be a delightful adventure for her. After getting her ears pierced, she joyfully posed for several pictures with two heavily tattooed staff members at the shop. She was thrilled with her new piercings and cherished the photographs from her memorable outing.

These examples demonstrate how caregivers can guide while respecting the individual's choices and autonomy.

8. Never Command or Demand, Instead Ask or Model:

Direct commands or demands can lead to confrontations. This story is a practical illustration of "Never Command or Demand." In one nursing home, a lovely lady, Judy, cherished a stuffed animal collection, which she affectionately called her "babies." She would often talk to them and proudly share stories about them with others.

During Easter, an incident highlighted the importance of understanding and compassion in caregiving. A family member of another resident brought in an Easter basket that contained a stuffed bunny. While they were visiting, the bunny was inadvertently left on a table. Judy, with her fondness for stuffed animals, noticed the bunny and immediately picked it up, drawing to it like her own collection.

Upon realizing the bunny was not hers, a caregiver attempted to retrieve it, telling her it was not her property. Unfortunately, this approach escalated into a confrontation. It was then that a more empathetic strategy was employed. The staff brought one of her own beloved 'babies' and proposed a trade. Judy was receptive to this idea and willingly exchanged the bunny for her stuffed animal.

The approach a caregiver or family member utilizes can avoid creating confrontations and maintain happiness and joy.

9. Never Condescend, Instead Encourage and Praise:

Bathing can often become a chore akin to climbing a mountain. Condescension can demean dementia patients, so avoid making them 'bad' for not bathing. Instead, emphasize creating a comfortable and enjoyable environment through methods like playing soothing music or providing soap in their favorite scent. This illustrates the importance of a respectful and encouraging approach. To support bathing, tell them how much you love them when they smell like those scents. If they complain that it is too cold (a common complaint), consider turning up the heat before bathtime, get a space heater, or try warming the towels. Create a spa experience and tell them, "We have spa day today!". Prepare everything in advance so your attention can be given to the bather. Praise and compliment them when finished.

10. Never Force, Instead Reinforce:

Forcing dementia patients to accept reality can be counterproductive. The case of the gentleman in the nursing home who periodically felt the need to go to work illustrates the importance of creative and empathetic approaches in caregiving, especially for individuals with dementia. This man was convinced he needed to go to work at least once a week. His sense of duty varied; sometimes, he believed he was in the Army, and other times, he thought he worked at a bank. It was crucial to handle his urges with care, as straightforwardly telling him he could not go would often lead to anger or even physical reactions, given his confusion and frustration.

The staff employed a thoughtful strategy when distraction was not effective. Another staff member would call him, posing as someone from his workplace, and inform him that work had been canceled for various reasons. They reassured him that he was excused for the day. This approach worked wonders; he would feel relieved and even pleased about not having to work, happily returning to bed.

A particularly touching moment was when the staff organized a retirement party for him. This event included guests, food, and a beautifully framed, large retirement certificate. This certificate was then displayed on the wall where he could see it. Whenever he noticed it, it helped him 'remember' that he was retired, easing his compulsion to go to work. This story underscores the significance of recognition and celebration in maintaining the patient's sense of identity and reality.

These principles emphasize the importance of empathy, understanding, and patience in dementia care. They advocate for approaches that respect the individual's experience and promote safety, dignity, and well-being.

As we continue to grow in our skills, let us move on to dementia behaviors and how to interpret them as a form of communication, further illuminating a path to deeper understanding and connection with those you care for.

3

The Art of Adaptation: Behavior Management in Dementia

Understanding the Shifts: Behavioral Changes in Dementia

Behavioral changes in a person with dementia can be diverse and challenging. Here are some key behavioral changes:

1. Repetitive Behavior:

People with dementia often repeat actions, words, or questions. This may be due to memory loss, where they cannot remember what they have done or said. Providing reassurance, distraction, or a calm response can be helpful.

2. Hiding, Hoarding, and Losing Things:

Individuals with dementia may hide or hoard items or frequently lose them, often because of memory loss. They might place items in unusual places or believe that items are being stolen. To assist, keep items in consistent places and consider using locator devices for frequently misplaced items. Ruth, living independently, was beginning to show memory loss symptoms and kept losing her purse. She accused others of taking it, but family members consistently found her wallet in the oven. Ruth soon needed more help and moved to a facility, but in the meantime, Ruth's family disconnected her stove for safety and told Ruth that the stove was broken and needed to be fixed. They also ensured she did not need to cook and helped her with meals.

3. Losing Inhibitions:

This can manifest as rudeness, inappropriate comments, or unusual behaviors like undressing in public. It often stems from changes in the brain and a lack of awareness of social norms. Managing this behavior involves patience, understanding, and protecting the individual's dignity. In one instance, in a facility, Connie had a manicure. She was so excited about how beautiful her nails looked that she came out of her room for dinner without any clothing. She commented to staff, holding up her hands to show off her fingernails, "I have never been so well dressed!" To maintain her dignity, staff members immediately took her back to her room to help her dress while commenting on her fabulous manicure.

4. Accusing:

Paranoia and delusions can lead to accusations, such as believing that items are stolen. It's important not to argue but to provide reassurance and address the underlying emotional need.

5. Agitation and Restlessness:

Agitation in dementia can include irritability, sleeplessness, and aggression, often due to environmental factors or changes in the brain. Creating a calm environment, maintaining routines, and providing soothing activities can be beneficial. Past jobs and responsibilities can influence the needs of dementia patients. Steve had been a city maintenance worker and was accustomed to being busy. As his dementia progressed, he became angry and combative, prompting his family to admit him to a nursing home. Knowing his history, the staff set up an area that needed 'work' to satisfy him. They asked Steve if he could help and gave him a paintbrush and a small water container. Making sure he was safe, he spent time happily 'painting,' frequently commenting on how much better the wall looked. His agitation decreased because he felt needed and felt that he was contributing.

6. Sleep disturbances and sundowning:

People with dementia may experience restlessness and agitation worsening in the evening (sundowning) and have trouble sleeping at night. Increasing daytime activities and reducing stimulants like caffeine can help.

7. Social Withdrawal:

A person with dementia may withdraw from activities or conversation. This could be due to difficulty in communicating or overwhelming situations. Providing opportunities for less stimulating activities can be helpful. Intimate, one-on-one interactions in a quiet, calm environment help make the person feel safe.

8. Aggressive Behavior:

may result from frustration, confusion, or environmental triggers. Ensuring safety and not confronting the person directly could be effective ways to manage aggression.

9. Wandering:

People with dementia may wander due to confusion, restlessness, or looking for something or someone. Measures such as locks or alarms may be necessary to ensure the safety of a person who may wander.

Caring for someone with dementia is a profoundly challenging journey. It can be heart-wrenching to see a loved one's personality and behaviors change so drastically. As a caregiver, you may face various emotions - frustration, sadness, confusion, and even guilt. These feelings are entirely normal and valid. Each day can bring new challenges as you navigate repetitive questions, agitation, paranoia, and other distressing behaviors. It is important to remember that your loved one's actions are symptoms of the disease, not a reflection of their character or your caregiving.

Despite these difficulties, your role is precious. Your patience, understanding, and compassion make a significant difference in your loved one's life. Remember, it is also essential to take care of yourself. Seek support from others in similar situations, and do not hesitate to seek professional help. Your strength and dedication, even in such challenges, are truly admirable.

Five Ground Rules to Consider in Managing Behaviour

Managing the behavioral changes of a loved one or patient with dementia requires understanding, patience, and a set of adaptable strategies. The Family Caregiver Alliance outlines five essential ground rules (Caregiver's Guide to Understanding Dementia Behaviors - Family Caregiver Alliance, 2022)

1. **We cannot change the person**: Recognize that dementia has altered the person's brain function, and trying to control or change their behavior is often futile. Instead, adapt your behavior and the environment to accommodate their needs.

2. **Check with the doctor first**: Before attributing all behavioral changes to dementia, consult a healthcare provider to rule out other medical reasons like pain, infection, or medication side effects. A UTI can quickly and dramatically change the emotions and behaviors of older individuals, so be sure to check with their physician if you have concerns.

3. **Behavior has a purpose**: People with dementia might be unable to express their needs or desires clearly. Their behavior, however perplexing, is often an attempt to fulfill a need. Try to identify and accommodate these underlying needs.

4. **Behavior is triggered**: All behavior has a trigger stemming from environmental factors, the actions of others, or internal states. Understanding and altering these triggers can help manage challenging behaviors.

5. **What works today may not work tomorrow**: The progressive nature of dementia means that effective strategies may need to change over time. Flexibility and creativity are key in adapting to new challenges and behaviors.

Use the questions below to help the caregiver understand and effectively respond to the behavioral changes in people with dementia. These questions can help identify causes of behavior changes, enabling the caregiver to strategize interventions to avoid the behaviors.

Guide Questions

1. What specific behavior did you observe, and in what context did it occur?
2. How does this behavior differ from the individual's usual behavior?
3. Are there any external factors that might be influencing this behavior?
4. What emotions or needs might be driving this behavior?
5. How does this behavior affect you as the caregiver?
6. What strategies have you tried in response to this behavior, and what were the outcomes?
7. Are there any environmental or routine changes that could help address this behavior?

Strategies For Managing Agitation, De-escalation, and Comfort

To manage agitation, de-escalation, and comfort in a person with dementia, consider these strategies:

1. Use the DICE Tool:

- **D: Describe what happens**: Observe and note the specifics of the behavior and its impact on both the patient and caregiver.
- **I: Investigate possible causes**: Look for underlying reasons such as medical conditions, environmental factors, or unmet needs.
- **C: Create a plan**: Develop strategies to address the behavior, considering the patient, caregiver, and environment.

- **E: Evaluate the plan**: Regularly assess the effectiveness of your approach and adjust as needed. (Behavior & Personality Changes, 2014)

2. Use Finesse, and Do Not be Afraid to Fudge the Truth: Be delicate and strategic in your approach. If the person with dementia becomes upset, apologizing, even if you are not at fault, can help defuse the situation. The goal is to maintain their dignity and comfort, not to prove a point.

3. Make Up a Story to Help Them Relax: Sometimes, creating a narrative can be calming. For instance, if they are worried about a non-existent appointment, you might reassure them that it has been rescheduled.

4. Don't Point Out Inaccurate or Strange Statements: Arguing or correcting them often increases confusion and agitation. It is better to go along with their reality as long as it is not harmful.

5. Keep Unsafe Items out of Sight: This helps prevent accidents or harmful behaviors.

6. Supervise Hygiene Routines: Assistance with daily tasks can prevent frustration and ensure safety.

7. Spend Time Together: Engaging in activities they enjoy can provide comfort and a sense of normalcy.

These strategies are not all-encompassing but can be effective starting points in managing complex behaviors associated with dementia. Everyone is different, so it is crucial to be flexible and adjust your approach as needed.

Making Sense of It All

A young nursing student, Mallory, working as a home health aide with profound insight into the caregiving journey, had this to say:

"After being a Certified Nursing Assistant for over three years, the most valuable lesson I have learned is that people with dementia are incredibly wise. When you sit and talk with them, you learn wonderful things about their perspective on life. I have found that the key to communicating with people who have this disease is to treat them like they have no condition that hinders them at all. When people talk down to those with dementia or other conditions and put limits on their abilities, it only makes things worse. People with dementia are often aware of it, and it can become very frustrating for them to try to find their way through their confusing thoughts.

It is important to keep their minds active, evident in a gentleman I cared for daily for two years. Even though he was constantly confused, I interacted with him like I had no idea he had dementia, which made a world of difference to him. I would take him to run errands and have him push the cart. I would do crafts with him and let him take all the time he needed to complete them. I took him to see Christmas lights, to coffee shops, to the movies, to the mall, and to play with my puppy. Whatever I could do to keep his mind active was the key to his happiness, and it was so inspiring to watch him live these things over and over like it was the first time.

If he got upset or frustrated, I would live that with him. If he noticed something out of the ordinary and was confused by it, instead of trying to over-explain or correct him, I would be curious about it with him. Having conversations about his concerns made him feel understood. I always tried to remember to live in whatever type of day he was having with him.

People with dementia are trying to figure things out, just like we are. Instead of losing patience, reassuring them that everything is okay is crucial. Answer their question patiently, as if it is the first time and not the eighth or twentieth time you have been asked. Divert the conversation if the topic is upsetting. Bring up the old days and good memories. Learn as much as you can to find out who they are as a person, where they were from, what experiences they have had, and who they love. These are the moments when reminiscing can create a deep and meaningful bond.

For me, I fell in love with the process of taking care of people with dementia. I fell in love with getting to know them again and again. I fell in love with becoming family and letting them know they are loved. I fell in love with reassuring them that everything is okay and they are perfect just how they are."

Mallory's insights serve as a beacon of empathy and understanding. Her experiences underscore the importance of seeing beyond the disease to the person within, creating a caregiving approach rooted in dignity, patience, and love.

By embracing practical, heart-centered skills, caregivers can enhance their effectiveness and forge deeper emotional connections, making each moment meaningful and filled with grace. Through the stories of Emma, Joel, and Mallory, we witness the profound impact of patience, adaptability, and innovative communication strategies on enhancing the quality of life for both caregivers and their loved ones.

As dementia alters the abilities of those we care for, it also invites us to grow, learn, and adapt alongside them. The journey is filled with challenges, yet it is also replete with opportunities for profound connection, learning, and personal growth. By approaching each day with empathy, understanding, and a willingness to meet our loved ones where they are, we can navigate the complexities of dementia with grace and resilience. This chapter is a testament to the power of compassionate care, offering both hope and practical guidance for those walking the caregiving path. It reminds us that, in the world of dementia care, our humanity, compassion, and resilience are our greatest assets.

Chapter 4 will illuminate the impact of patience and empathy on both the caregiver and the person with dementia, emphasizing that these virtues enhance our care and nurture an environment where understanding and compassion prevail. As we move to this next chapter, prepare to embrace the power of patience and empathy and learn how they become our strongest allies in the journey of dementia caregiving.

4

Patience and Empathy

The Twin Pillars of Effective Caregiving

I n the heart of every caregiver lies a story of love, resilience, and profound dedication. Yet, during the daily challenges of dementia care, even the most steadfast hearts can find themselves searching for sustenance. This chapter is a lighthouse of hope and guidance, illuminating the path to nurturing two of the most essential virtues in caregiving: patience and empathy. Here, we delve into the transformative power of these qualities, not just as mere concepts but as practical, daily practices that can intensely reshape your caregiving experience. Through insightful strategies and compassionate understanding, we will explore how patience and empathy can become your steadfast allies, turning everyday moments into opportunities for deep connection and mutual growth. Whether you are a seasoned caregiver or just beginning this journey, these pages promise to enrich your understanding and empower you with tools that bring out the best in you and your loved one, making every day a testament to the strength and beauty of the human spirit.

This chapter continues with Step 2, emphasizing the 'A' in C.A.R.E.S.S., which also stands for Adaptation through developing patience and empathy. This step is a cornerstone in our journey, as it guides caregivers on how to adapt their approach and mindset to connect with and support their loved ones effectively. By embracing and cultivating patience and empathy, caregivers can navigate the often complex and unpredictable landscape of dementia care with greater ease and understanding.

As we embark on the journey through the chapter, let us begin with a profound thought from the esteemed Leo Tolstoy: "Patience is waiting. Not passively waiting. That is laziness. But to keep going when the going is hard and slow - that is patience." This insightful quote resonates deeply with the essence of caregiving, especially in the context of dementia.

In this chapter, we will see that patience in caregiving isn't about a resigned acceptance of hardship but rather a resilient, ongoing commitment to care, even when progress seems elusive. This form of patience is a proactive force, driving us to adapt, learn, and grow alongside our loved ones. Furthermore, we will intertwine the concept of empathy with patience, understanding how these two virtues amplify each other, creating a more compassionate and effective caregiving environment.

Empathy allows us to understand the world of our loved ones, which in turn fuels our patience as we become more attuned to their needs and challenges. This chapter discusses these concepts and provides practical strategies and real-life examples to cultivate these qualities in our daily caregiving journey.

The Heart of Patience: A Deeper Look into Caregiving

Patience in dementia caregiving involves tolerating delays, troubles, or suffering without becoming angry or upset. This quality is crucial in dementia care as it often consists of overcoming various challenges, including the overwhelming demands of prolonged caregiving, safety issues, repetition, slowness, loss of ability to do simple things, and personality changes in the person with dementia (Patience - the Center for Brain/Mind Medicine, 2022).

Cultivating a mindset of patience is beneficial for both the caregiver and the person with dementia. However, it's essential to acknowledge that being patient at all times is nearly impossible, especially as dementia is one of the most challenging medical conditions (Heltemes, 2016). Maintaining a positive tone and outlook can help smooth interactions and prevent behaviors that may later be regretted. Frustration is a common byproduct of the challenging work of caregiving, making patience a vital component of providing person-centered care that focuses on comfort, dignity, and quality of life (Connolly, 2021).

Why Patience Matters: Uncovering its Significance in Dementia Care

Patience in caregiving involves adapting to the changing needs and abilities of the person with dementia. Caregivers are encouraged to step back and assess situations calmly, responding thoughtfully rather than reacting impulsively. This approach includes understanding that the person with dementia may experience time shifts or hallucinations, and rather than correcting these perceptions, caregivers should seek to connect by engaging in conversations about these experiences. Activities and plans should be flexible, prioritizing the emotional needs and dignity of the person with dementia.

Patience is essential in caring for individuals with dementia for several reasons. Let us discuss them one by one:

1. **Communication Becomes More Difficult**. Dementia affects a person's ability to communicate effectively. Caregivers need to be patient and thoughtful in their interactions, recognizing that communication challenges are symptoms of their condition. They should consider nonverbal cues and be prepared to enter the person's reality, especially if they are experiencing hallucinations or time traveling. Engaging the senses in visual, verbal, and touch cues can help communication.

2. **Performing Daily Tasks Takes More Time**. People with dementia often require more time to complete everyday activities. Caregivers must adjust their expectations and plans accordingly, understanding that tasks like eating or showering may take longer than usual. It is important to maintain the dignity and respect of the person with dementia, accommodating their pace and emotional needs.

3. **Behavior and Personality Changes Occur**: Dementia can cause significant changes in behavior and personality. Caregivers must learn to adapt to these changes, getting new ways to communicate and cooperate with the person. This might involve altering activities to suit their changing abilities or finding creative ways to engage them. It is also crucial for caregivers to take care of themselves, as the role can be emotionally and physically demanding.

Mastering Patience: Proven Techniques for Caregivers

Caregivers often find themselves managing one crisis after another, which can lead to high levels of stress and burnout. Caregivers who cultivate patience provide better care and maintain their mental and emotional happiness. Patience in dementia caregiving is a critical expertise that can be upgraded through mindfulness practices and practical caregiving strategies (Three Mindfulness Exercises to Reduce Caregiver Stress, 2017). Let's discuss them in detail:

1. Practice Mindfulness and Meditation

At its core, mindfulness is the art of staying anchored in the present moment, gently acknowledging our thoughts and emotions to help us relax and build emotional calm. This grounding technique proves invaluable in managing the rollercoaster of caregiver emotions.

- **Mindfulness Meditation**: This fundamental practice invites you to find a peaceful spot, sit comfortably, and close your eyes. Begin by taking deep, deliberate breaths, inhaling through the nose, and exhaling through the mouth. After a few breaths, let your breathing return to normal. You then engage in a 'body scan,' where you consciously observe your five senses, one by one. Notice the touch, smell, taste, sounds, and finally, what you see around you. This activity, which can be shared with your loved one, is a powerful way to connect and find peace during a stressful routine.
- **I Wish You Peace (Loving-Kindness Meditation)**: This meditation is about sending compassionate thoughts to yourself and others. It starts with finding a comfortable

spot and closing your eyes. First, you direct compassion towards yourself with affirmations like "May I be happy, well, and free from harm." You then extend these wishes to others: someone you love, a neutral person, someone you struggle with, and finally, everyone in the world. This practice of universal compassion can profoundly shift your perspective and bring a sense of peace and connectedness.

- **Gratitude Practice**: This exercise focuses on daily life's minor, often overlooked blessings. Keeping a dedicated journal for this purpose can be helpful. Here, you jot down anything that sparks a sense of gratitude—a joke, a memory, a small act of kindness. This practice is particularly beneficial in challenging times as a remembrance of the positive aspects of your life, thus fostering a sense of well-being and peace of mind.

People often feel they have difficulty 'quieting' their minds enough to gain benefits from meditation. Don't give up. Start with 5-10 minutes of meditation. As thoughts enter your mind, simply notice them, and let them go. As more thoughts enter your mind, let them go as well. As you gain proficiency, you will notice fewer and fewer thoughts interrupting your meditation. Whether you feel successful or not, practicing meditation will help you to become more self-aware and more patient, reduce negative feelings, and be able to manage stress more easily.

2. Communicate Clearly and Patiently

Clear and patient communication is vital when caring for someone with dementia. It is crucial to use simple, straightforward language and give the person time to process and respond. For example, instead of saying, "Do you recall what we did yesterday?" you might ask, "Did you enjoy the music we listened to yesterday?"

This direct approach reduces confusion and helps maintain a connection despite memory challenges.

3. Take Breaks When Needed

Caregiving is demanding, and regular breaks are essential for maintaining mental and physical health. Whether it is a short walk, reading a book, or a weekend getaway, these breaks help prevent caregiver burnout. For instance, taking a daily 20-minute walk can help clear your mind and reduce stress.

4. Remember It is Not Personal

It is important to remember that a person with dementia's challenging behaviors, like anger or confusion, are symptoms, not personal attacks. Understanding this can help caregivers manage their emotional responses more effectively. When your loved one becomes upset, remind yourself that it is the dementia speaking, not them.

5. Join a Support Group

Assistance groups offer a room for caregivers to share experiences, offer advice, and gain emotional support. For instance, an online support group can provide tips on managing daily challenges and a platform to express feelings in a safe, understanding environment.

6. Set Small, Realistic Goals

Setting small, achievable goals can make caregiving more manageable and give a sense of accomplishment. For example, setting a goal to walk or do chair yoga for 15 minutes with your loved one daily can be realistic and beneficial for both of you.

7. Use Engaging Activities

Incorporating engaging activities like music, exercise, and art can significantly increase the worth of life for someone with dementia. Music, for example, can trigger memories and positive emotions. Simple exercises, such as gentle walks, can maintain physical health, while art activities like painting offer a creative channel and a sense of completion. Chair yoga is a wonderful alternative for exercise, even if the person is not ambulatory, and a beneficial practice for caregivers.

8. Avoid Over-Stimulation and Stick to Routines

People with dementia often thrive on routine and can become quickly exhausted by too much stimulus. Keeping a consistent daily schedule and avoiding noisy, crowded environments can help reduce anxiety and confusion. A calm, structured day can provide a sense of security.

9. Learn About the Disease

Understanding dementia is critical to providing effective care. This knowledge can help anticipate needs, manage symptoms, and communicate effectively. For example, learning about the progression of dementia can help you understand why your loved one's abilities and behaviors change over time.

10. Try Humor and Laughter

Humor and laughter can be powerful tools in caregiving. They help relieve stress and can create joyful moments. For example, sharing a funny story or watching a comedy together can lighten the mood and consolidate the link between caregiver and loved one.

In summary, these strategies encompass a holistic approach to dementia caregiving, focusing on effective communication, self-care, understanding the nature of the disease, and incorporating enjoyable activities. They are designed not just to manage the challenges of dementia care but to enhance the quality of life for both the caregiver and the person they care for (Caregiver Stress, 2024).

Empathy: The Invisible Bridge in Dementia Care

Empathy in dementia care involves the ability to deeply understand and share the feelings and experiences of a person with dementia. As Alzheimer's disease, including other types of dementia, progresses, individuals may find it increasingly difficult to express themselves verbally. Consequently, they may communicate their feelings and needs through behaviors such as resistance to assistance or becoming overwhelmed in specific environments. The Validation Method, developed by social worker Naomi Feil, embodies this empathetic approach. It involves stepping into the world of the person with dementia, mirroring their emotions, and using open questions to help them express their feelings (Using Empathy to Care for a Loved One with Alzheimer's, 2019).

Empathy is fundamentally about putting oneself in another's shoes and feeling what they feel. In dementia care, this means understanding the rapidly changing behaviors and emotions the condition can cause (Brandon, 2017) . Empathetic caregiving enhances communication, particularly with those who struggle to articulate their thoughts and reduces feelings of loneliness or isolation in dementia patients.

Remember, caregivers must also be mindful of their mental health. Emotional burnout can occur without proper self-care and boundaries, which may diminish the caregiver's capacity for empathy. Caregivers should engage in active listening and empathetic reflection to cultivate empathy effectively and seek education and training in compassionate caregiving if needed. Regular breaks, joining support groups, and setting personal boundaries are crucial for caregivers to maintain their emotional well-being and empathy (Empathy in Caregiving, 2023).

Empathetic caregiving offers care that addresses the emotional and psychological well-being of the person with dementia. It can also inspire others in the community or family to act with similar compassion, fostering a supportive environment for all. Ultimately, empathy in caregiving enhances the quality of care and enriches the caregiver's experience, enabling deeper connections and gratification in their role.

Empathy in Action: Why It's Essential in Dementia Care

Empathy stands at the heart of effective dementia care, serving as a vital bridge between caregivers and those living with dementia. It goes beyond mere understanding, allowing caregivers to connect deeply with individuals who may struggle to communicate their experiences and needs due to cognitive impairments. By empathetically engaging with patients, caregivers can navigate the complexities of dementia with compassion and understanding, ultimately enriching the lives of those they care for. The act of empathy has many reasons, some of them are:

1. Building Trust and Emotional Bonds:

Establishing trust and emotional bonds is critical in dementia care. When caregivers employ empathy, they acknowledge the unique perspective of the person with dementia. The caregiver fosters a sense of safety and understanding by engaging in active, compassionate listening and responding to non-verbal cues. This approach builds trust, as the person with dementia feels genuinely heard and valued, creating a stronger emotional bond between caregiver and patient.

2. Understanding Unspoken Feelings:

Due to cognitive impairments, individuals with dementia often struggle to communicate their feelings verbally. Empathy allows caregivers to pick up on subtle non-verbal cues and changes in behavior, providing insights into the unspoken emotions and needs of a person with dementia. With no disrespect to those with dementia, it is much like how we anticipate the needs of babies before they can communicate with words. By tuning into these silent signals, caregivers can respond more effectively to the person's emotional state, ensuring their needs are met even when they cannot articulate them.

3. Reducing Caregiver Stress:

Understanding the patient's perspective helps caregivers make sense of challenging behaviors, leading to less frustration and a more fulfilling caregiving experience. This empathetic approach reduces stress and burnout, enhancing the caregiver's ability to provide consistent, high-quality care.

4. Enhancing Patient Health Outcomes:

Empathy directly impacts the health outcomes of individuals with dementia. When caregivers respond empathetically to their needs, patients often exhibit reduced anxiety and agitation, improving overall well-being. Empathetic care can also enhance the effectiveness of other treatments and interventions, as patients feel more comfortable and cooperative in a supportive and understanding environment.

5. Connecting with Patients' Loved Ones:

Empathy extends beyond the caregiver-patient relationship to include the patient's loved ones. By demonstrating understanding and compassion, caregivers can form meaningful connections with family members, offering them support and reassurance. This approach helps families navigate the challenges of dementia care, creating a supportive network for both the patient and their loved ones.

6. Managing Emotions:

Dementia care can be emotionally overwhelming for both the caregiver and the patient. By recognizing and validating the feelings of the person with dementia, caregivers can alleviate distress and confusion. Simultaneously, empathetic self-awareness allows caregivers to acknowledge and address their emotional responses, maintaining their mental health and resilience in the face of challenging caregiving situations.

Cultivating Empathy: A Caregiver's Guide to Enhanced Interactions

Empathy, a fundamental tool in dementia care, requires understanding and feeling the world as the person with dementia does. It is about stepping into their shoes, recognizing the challenges in communication as the disease progresses, and employing strategies like the Validation Method to address behavioral expressions. Empathy training emphasizes skills such as reading body language, avoiding judgments, and appreciating the unique experiences of each individual. Empathy workshops provide practical insights, simulating the sensory and cognitive impairments of dementia, thereby deepening caregivers' understanding and enhancing their ability to connect with and support those living with dementia.

Empathy workshops, like the one conducted by Samvedna Care, use experiential activities to foster a deeper understanding of the dementia experience. For instance, participants might undergo simulations that mimic the sensory and cognitive impairments of dementia, such as vision and hearing alterations, to appreciate the daily challenges those with the condition face. This immersive approach enhances empathy and sheds light on the importance of non-verbal communication in late-stage dementia care (Samvedna, 2017).

Here are strategies emphasizing the importance of empathy, patience, and understanding in dementia care. These strategies are collected from different resources, including Communication and Alzheimer's (2024), Brandon (2017), and Using Empathy to Care for a Loved One with Alzheimer's (2019).

1. Listen Actively:

To actively listen means giving full attention to the person with dementia. Retain eye contact and use spoken signals like "I see" or "I understand" to show you are engaged and listening. This approach helps in understanding their needs and emotions.

2. Validate Their Feelings:

Acknowledging and validating their emotions is crucial. Use statements like "I understand this must be frustrating" or "I can see you are feeling sad right now" to validate their feelings. This helps them feel heard and understood.

3. Use Positive Language:

Avoid negative words like "No," "don't," and "can't," which can be discouraging. Instead, use positive language such as "Yes," "do," and "can" to encourage and support them.

4. Be Patient:

Patience is vital in dementia care. Tolerate delays, confusion, or repetitive statements with compassion, understanding that these are part of the condition.

5. Provide Reassurance:

Offer reassurance to convey support, even if their concerns seem irrational. Phrases like "I'm here for you," or a simple hand squeeze can be very comforting.

6. Engage Their Senses Through Music, Art, Pets, and Other Sensory Outlets:

Respond to their behavioral expressions using tools like touch, music, nature, and art. These can have profound benefits in connecting with them and providing comfort.

7. Reminisce Positive Memories:

Tapping into memories still impactful for the person with dementia can be a powerful way to connect and bring joy. It helps in maintaining a sense of identity and personal history. Look at old photos or mementos to help connect with those memories.

8. Involve Loved Ones to Foster Social Bonds and Relationships:

It is important to keep the person with dementia involved in social activities and conversations. This maintains their sense of belonging and social bonds.

A Symphony of Empathy and Patience: Enriching Your Caregiving Journey

In caregiving, particularly for those with dementia, the interplay of patience and empathy emerges as a cornerstone for effective care. The following ideas from (Robin, 2023), (DeAngelis, 2023), and (Nasir, 2023) delve into the profound impact these qualities have on both the caregiver and the person with dementia.

1. For Someone with Dementia:

- **Person-Centered Care Respectful, Compassionate, and Tailored**

Patience allows caregivers to understand and meet the unique needs of everyone with dementia. By taking time to understand their history, preferences, and routines, caregivers can provide personalized care that respects the person's autonomy and identity.

Empathy helps in recognizing and validating the emotions of the person with dementia. Empathy fosters a deep connection, making them feel heard and understood, thereby enhancing their sense of self-worth and belonging.

- **Reduced Distress**

Caregivers who approach situations with patience are less likely to escalate distressing situations. Patience helps caregivers calmly navigate challenging behaviors or communication barriers, thereby reducing anxiety and agitation in dementia patients.

By empathetically acknowledging their fears and frustrations, caregivers can provide comfort, making the person with dementia feel safer and more secure.

- **Enhanced Trust, Dignity, Comfort, and Well-being**

Create a nurturing environment where the person with dementia feels valued and respected. This enhances their trust in the caregiver, fostering a sense of dignity and overall well-being. A comforting presence and understanding attitude help alleviate feelings of isolation and confusion.

2. For Caregivers:

- **More Fulfillment and Better Outcomes**

Empathy leads to a deeper connection with the person cared for, making caregiving more rewarding. Understanding the person's life story and experiences enriches the caregiving experience. Meanwhile, patience allows for developing effective strategies tailored to the individual's needs, leading to more successful outcomes and a sense of achievement.

- **Prevent Burnout**

Patience helps manage expectations and accept the progressive nature of dementia. Recognizing that some days will be challenging enables caregivers to approach caregiving with a balanced perspective, reducing the risk of burnout.

- **Improved Communication**

Patience in communication involves allowing time for the person with dementia to express themselves, even if communication is non-verbal. Being patient in interpreting their needs and responses fosters better understanding. Empathetic listening involves truly hearing and trying to understand what the person with dementia is attempting to communicate, which is crucial for effective care and emotional support.

- **Reduced Caregiver Depression and Anxiety**

Recognizing the emotional challenges and the unpredictability of dementia can help caregivers manage their expectations and emotions. Additionally, accepting that there will be good and bad days helps in maintaining a more stable emotional state, reducing feelings of depression and anxiety.

- **Enhanced Caregiver Competence**

Caregiving for someone with dementia is a learning process. Patience helps in gradually acquiring the skills and knowledge necessary for effective caregiving. On the other hand, empathy can guide decision-making, ensuring that the care provided is in the best interest of the person with dementia, thereby enhancing the caregiver's sense of competence. When you give care with the best interest of the person with dementia always foremost in mind, you can rest assured that you are doing the right thing.

This chapter emphasizes the critical roles of patience and empathy in effective dementia caregiving. It highlights that patience is not just about enduring difficulties but about adapting to the evolving needs of someone with dementia. This adaptation is crucial due to the progressive nature of dementia, affecting communication, daily task performance, and behavior. In this chapter, we suggest practical strategies for caregivers to cultivate patience with mindfulness practices, straightforward communication tips, and self-care strategies like taking breaks, joining support groups, and, most importantly, setting realistic goals. Practicing these strategies will help to reduce caregiver stress, ultimately improving the quality of care.

Empathy, on the other hand, is about deeply understanding and sharing the feelings of a person with dementia. It is essential for building trust, enhancing patient health outcomes, and reducing caregiver stress. We provided guidance on developing empathy with active listening, positive language, and engaging the patient's senses. The combination of empathy and patience in caregiving leads to person-centered care, reduced stress for the patient, and a more fulfilling, less stressful experience for the caregiver. This approach not only improves communication and outcomes but also helps prevent caregiver burnout, depression, and anxiety, enhancing overall satisfaction and happiness for all parties.

In chapter five, we will use techniques to support the caregiver in further developing and maintaining patience and empathy in their demanding role while cultivating the resilience to thrive.

You can Make a Difference

There's a magical thing about giving-it helps the one who receives and brings joy to the giver.

> *"Everyone can experience the joy and blessings of generosity because everyone has something to give."*

> Jan Grace

What if you could extend a hand and be a blessing to someone in need? Maybe someone is looking for guidance in their dementia journey.

People choose books based on their cover and, more importantly, what others say about them. This book can reach more readers seeking help with reviews from people like you.

If you are finding value in "Dementia Support for Caregivers and Families", a heartfelt review about how this book has touched you and why you think it may be valuable for other caregivers and families may be the lifeline of hope and guidance they need.

My mission is to make "Dementia Support for Caregivers and Families" a beacon of hope for everyone. So, I'm kindly asking for your assistance on behalf of the many dementia caregivers and families out there looking for a helping hand:

Would you leave an honest review? It takes less than a minute, and the words you share could be the key to unlocking the world of empathy, strategies, and support for someone struggling with dementia care.

Please, help me reach those in need. Together, we can build a bridge of support and understanding one review at a time. Your contribution is more than just words: it's a lifeline of hope and guidance for someone in need.

You can leave a quick review by scanning the QR code below. Thank you for sharing your thoughts and contributing to the lives of others.

Now back to the topic at hand...

Your biggest fan,
Hanna Wells

From Stress to Strength

Building Emotional Resilience in the Face of Dementia

In many homes, a silent and emotional journey happens every day. It is a path filled with love, sacrifice, and the hidden challenges of caring for someone with dementia. This chapter invites you to recognize and accept the emotions that come with this vital role. We will look closely at what it really means to care for someone with dementia. You will learn about the stresses and challenges and the incredible chances for personal growth and emotional strength. We will move from feeling emotionally overwhelmed to becoming resilient, showing the strength of the human spirit in tough times. Together, we will discover practical tips and heartfelt advice, helping caregivers and families get by and thrive, even during one of life's most difficult challenges.

Chapter 5 will identify stressors to understand our emotional well-being and learn strategies and exercises to build resilience. Mastery of these skills will make a positive impact in every area of your life.

Before we delve into the core of his chapter, let us pause to focus on a pivotal element of the C.A.R.E.S.S. Method, Step 3: Resilience. This step is the cornerstone around which our strategies and insights revolve. Resilience, in the context of dementia caregiving, is not just about enduring; it is about the ability to continually adapt and thus thrive during the complexities and emotional rollercoaster this journey entails. In the following pages, we will explore how to cultivate this resilience, transforming it from a mere concept into a tangible, daily practice. This is where we learn to balance the scales between the weight of our responsibilities and the strength of our emotional and mental well-being. As we embark on this crucial part of our journey, remember that resilience is not a quality we are born with but a skill we can build with a prize that will ultimately benefit ourselves and our families in the face of dementia.

Statistics show that nearly 75% of dementia caregivers worry about their health deterioration amidst their demanding roles. Further intensifying this concern, over one-third of these care-givers acknowledge a decline in their health due to their care-giving responsibilities. These statistics emphasize the importance of caregivers being proactive about their own physical health and emotional wellness. This chapter explores strategies to build emotional resilience and maintain overall health, offering guid-ance and support in navigating these turbulent waters (Caregiver Statistics: Health, Technology, and Caregiving Resources – Family Caregiver Alliance, 2016).

Take Glenda, for instance, who has been caring for her mother for five years. Here is what she has to say about her caregiving journey:

"At first, my mom was still living independently, and my visits were focused on routine tasks like ensuring she made it to appointments and paid bills on time. These early days were manageable and enjoyable for both of us. However, as her ability to perform daily tasks began to decline, my visits became more frequent to assist with household chores and cooking.

The situation became more challenging when my mom started misplacing items in unusual spots, such as putting her purse in the dishwasher. Attempts to correct her only led to frustration on both sides, highlighting the progression of her dementia and signaling the need for a change.

When I moved her into my home, I sought support from our family and her doctor, which helped in decision-making. My brother's involvement provided me with some much-needed personal time. We educated ourselves on dementia and improved our communication methods. Establishing a Durable Power of Attorney and tackling financial planning alleviated many concerns.

A significant shift occurred when I began implementing the "10 Absolutes". I realized that my well-intentioned corrections were making my mom feel invalidated. Adopting a more acceptable approach, where I met her in her reality, transformed our lives; she became happier and more engaged, living with dignity despite the tough days.

Reflecting on this journey, I'm deeply grateful for the experience of caring for my mom. It has enriched my life, allowing me to love and find joy in every day with her, even as we deal with the challenges of dementia. Our time together is precious, and I treasure every moment."

Unraveling the Mystery of Emotional Resilience

Emotional resilience in caregiving is a multifaceted concept vital for coping with the challenging aspects of caring for someone with chronic or advanced illness. It is defined as a positive outcome in the face of adversity and stress, characterized by an ability to adjust to experiences perceived as threatening (Palacio et al., 2019). This means you gain resilience by practicing the ability to adapt until you achieve the desired positive outcome. Just as Glenda had the resilience to adapt to changes with her mother, you, too, can experience caregiving with a new level of competence, ease, and joy. By its nature, caregiving often evokes a broad spectrum of positive and negative emotions. These feelings may emerge immediately or over time and include a mix of love, duty, fear, and frustration. Caregivers are sometimes reluctant to share negative emotions for fear of judgment or not wanting to burden others (The Emotional Side of Caregiving Family Caregiver Alliance, 2014).

However, caregivers must acknowledge and deal with these emotions, as ignoring them can lead to adverse effects like poor sleep and difficulty coping, which could lead to a variety of illnesses. Caregivers can manage their emotional well-being more effectively by acknowledging and expressing feelings productively. Research highlights the importance of self-care and the ability to derive positive experiences from caregiving in maintaining mental health and resilience. Acknowledging your frustrations and negative feelings along with your wins and celebrating the small victories in daily care is vital. This form of resilience enables caregivers to adapt to challenging situations and grow from them. Therefore, emotional resilience in caregiving involves recognizing and addressing the wide range of emotions that come with the role and developing coping strategies that promote well-being and adaptation (Trudy, 2021).

Dementia caregiving often involves a long-term commitment demanding both physical and emotional endurance from the caregiver, further underscoring the importance of developing your emotional resilience. The importance of resilience includes the following reasons:

1. Avoiding Burnout

Burnout typically arises from prolonged exposure to stress without adequate coping mechanisms, leading to physical, mental, and emotional exhaustion. By fostering resilience, caregivers can better manage the relentless demands of their role, thus mitigating feelings of being overwhelmed. Resilient caregivers are more likely to engage in self-care practices, set healthy boundaries, and seek support when needed, all of which are essential strategies to avoid burnout.

Consider for yourself:

- What is my current level of stress? Am I feeling burnt out?
- Do I do enough to take care of myself?
- Am I able to say no to others for my well-being?
- Who can I call on when I need help?

2. Navigating Emotional Challenges

Caregiving inevitably involves a range of emotional challenges, including feelings of frustration, guilt, sadness, and isolation. Emotional resilience equips caregivers to recognize, understand, and process these complex feelings effectively. It involves developing coping strategies that allow caregivers to navigate these emotional waters with more ease, thereby maintaining their emotional well-being while providing care.

Consider for yourself:

- Do I have a person or place where I can share my emotions, just vent, and get advice?
- Where else can I find a safe sharing platform?

3. Mental and Physical Health

The link between emotional resilience and caregivers' mental and physical health is significant. High resilience is associated with lower levels of stress, anxiety, and depression, contributing to better overall mental health. Moreover, resilient caregivers are more likely to maintain healthy lifestyles, engage in physical activity, and seek medical care as needed, which directly benefits their physical health. This holistic approach to health is crucial for sustaining the energy and stamina required for caregiving.

Consider for yourself:

- Do I exercise and eat a healthy diet?
- Do I have regular health checkups and follow my doctor's directions?
- What ways can I improve my physical health?

4. Flexibility in the Face of Change

Caregiving situations are dynamic and often unpredictable, requiring high flexibility. Emotional resilience enhances a caregiver's ability to adapt to changing circumstances, whether a sudden decline in the care recipient's health or a change in available resources. This adaptability is vital for effectively managing new challenges and minimizing change-related stress.

Consider for yourself:

- Do I consider myself flexible? Can I be more adaptable?
- Are there situations in caregiving that are more stressful than others to me?
- Can I arrange for help to support my emotional resilience?

5. Discovering Purpose and Growth

Emotional resilience can lead caregivers to discover a more profound sense of purpose and personal growth. When navigated successfully, caregiving challenges can foster a sense of accomplishment, strengthen personal values, and provide new insights into life. This perspective shift often leads caregivers to find meaning in their role and view their experiences as opportunities for growth and development. "Too often we underestimate the power of touch, a smile, a kind word, a listening ear, an honest compliment, or the smallest act of caring, all of which have the potential to turn a life around" (Buscaglia, A-Z Quotes, 2024). These small acts of caring that create positive outcomes for the person you care for are reasons for celebration and recognition of success. Acknowledge all your wins.

Consider for yourself:

- Do I give myself credit for every win in caregiving?
- Do I practice gratitude daily?
- Do I make a difference/bring happiness in the life of the person I care for?

6. Building Confidence and Competence

Finally, emotional resilience is instrumental in building confidence and competence in caregiving. Resilient caregivers develop a sense of mastery over their responsibilities, leading to confidence in their caregiving skills. This self-assurance, coupled with continued learning and adaptation, enhances their competence in providing care. As caregivers become more proficient, their resilience is further reinforced, creating a positive feedback loop that values both the caregiver and the care recipient.

Consider for yourself:

- What areas could I improve to develop my emotional resilience skills further?
- What area of caregiving am I most proficient in?

Caregivers can use this exercise to help them understand their current resilience level and identify improvement areas. Continuous reflection on and practice of resiliency through self-care practices, setting boundaries, and seeking support when needed will continue to strengthen your ability to cope with the daily struggles of caregiving and reach the point of mastery while thriving in the chaos and ever-changing world of dementia. Now, let's look deeper into the emotional challenges dementia caregivers face.

When Dementia Hits Home: Understanding it is Emotional Impact

The emotional challenges faced by dementia caregivers are profound and complex. Most of the time, caregivers face a range of intense emotions stemming from the demanding nature of their role. Feelings of frustration at the loved one's diminishing abilities and social withdrawal due to the all-consuming nature of their role are normal and understandable (Caregiver Stress, 2024). The unpredictable progression of dementia presents additional emotional burdens, as caregivers must constantly adapt to new symptoms and behaviors in their loved ones. This constant flux can be profoundly disorienting and emotionally draining (What Are the Main Challenges Faced by Dementia Caregivers? 2022).

Many caregivers describe feeling overwhelmed, anxious, and unable to perform daily tasks effectively due to the stress of their role. Moreover, the stress of caregiving can also lead to significant health issues, like cardiovascular disease, diabetes, insomnia, and stomach ulcers, further compounding the emotional challenges they face (Aaron, 2004). Failure to identify and address their ability to cope can leave caregivers susceptible to illness. The emotional health of caregivers for individuals with dementia is significantly impacted by their responsibilities and the nature of the illness they are dealing with (Caregiver Well-Being, 2024). We have learned that cultivating patience and empathy helps to ease caregiver tension. Building emotional resilience gives access to long-term empowerment, greatly helping to avoid the emotional and physical issues below, often caused by the stress of caregiving.

1. Loneliness and Social Isolation

The demanding nature of caregiving can limit opportunities for social interaction, leading to feeling cut off from the outside world. Friends may visit less frequently, and caregivers spend less time and energy maintaining social connections. As social life diminishes, the increased segregation can enhance feelings of loneliness and emotional distress for the caregiver.

Maintaining social connections with people or groups that support your well-being is a priority. Schedule regular times for social interaction with people who empower and support you emotionally. Stay connected. Having a group of people who can relate is essential. Enlarge your group if needed. Go out with your friends, go to family cookouts, and holiday dinners, go to church, to your support groups, or do whatever keeps you engaged.

2. Stress Hormones and Immune Function

The constant demands and stressors associated with caregiving can cause increased levels of stress hormones like cortisol. Have you ever noticed how you catch a cold when you are stressed? Increasing stress hormones is like constantly keeping the body's alarm system on. This can make it more likely to catch any infection or get sick because the immune system is busy fighting these stress signals.

3. Anxiety and Loss of Sleep

The stress of caregiving and witnessing a loved one's decline can trigger anxiety and depression. Caregivers constantly worry about the future and stream of caregiving tasks, making relaxing difficult. Disturbed sleep habits can lead to increased anxiety, emotional exhaustion, and depression.

Are you experiencing joy in caregiving? Laughter has great power. Laughter creates positive physiological changes in our bodies. Look for humor. Try not to take everything seriously and learn to laugh at yourself.

4. Anger, Resentment, and Frustration

These emotions often arise from the challenges of dealing with the loved one's declining abilities and the resulting increased dependence. Caregivers might feel anger towards their situation or resentment towards other family members who are not contributing enough. These types of emotions add another level of emotional stress.

When anxious or upset, practice relaxation and meditation techniques to find calm. Look for things or people that you are grateful for. Practice gratitude for all the good things in your life. Practice communicating your resentments without anger. Forgive yourself and others.

5. Ambiguous Loss, Grief and Loss of Control of Life

As dementia progresses, caregivers mourn the loss of the person they once knew, even though they are still physically present. This ambiguous loss is a profound source of grief and can be more challenging to cope with than a definitive loss like death.

Caregivers may miss having time for themselves and feel like they are not achieving much. This loss of life, as they knew it, is also something to grieve.

It is expected to grieve what we have lost. Do you need support to help you through the stages of grieving? Contact friends, family, support groups, or professionals like ministers for support.

6. Guilt and Helplessness

Most caregivers struggle with feelings of guilt and helplessness, questioning whether they are doing enough or making the right decisions. These feelings are often compounded by the progressive nature of dementia, where, despite their best efforts, the loved one's condition continues to deteriorate.

Seeking help and support from others is a vital part of caring for yourself. Do not hesitate to ask for what you need to support your mental and emotional health. This will encourage building resilience, keeping you emotionally and physically stronger. Sometimes, caregivers may not even know what they need for support. This is where peer groups are particularly helpful because they have had or are having the same experiences.

7. Difficulty Managing Behavioral Changes

Dementia can cause significant changes in behavior, such as agitation, anxiety, and apathy. Caregivers must continually adapt to these changes, often without clear guidance or support, which can be incredibly challenging and stressful. Using the techniques and methods in "Dementia Support for Caregivers and Families," you can learn to be flexible and creative while having fun and caring for your loved ones.

To all caregivers experiencing these challenges: Your feelings are valid, and you are not alone. Most caregivers have experienced some or all of these emotions and worries. Being a caregiver for someone with dementia is challenging and requires resilience. It is not just about the physical work but also the emotional weight. That is why it is vital to have good support and resources to help you navigate these complex emotions. It enables you to take care of yourself while caring for someone else. Remember, even superheroes need a helping hand sometimes!

Strategies to Develop Emotional Resilience

Caring for someone with Alzheimer's disease or dementia is a journey that requires not just love and patience but also a strategic approach to managing the inherent challenges and stress. In the following, we will discuss the methods for caregivers to navigate their responsibilities, drawing upon the collective wisdom of "Reducing Caregiver Stress" (2022), Ducharme (2018), and Sheehan et al. (2020). These steps empower caregivers with the tools necessary to maintain their well-being while providing the best possible care.

Step 1: Assess Your Caregiving Duties and Responsibilities

The first step in this journey is to assess your caregiving duties comprehensively. Begin by listing all your tasks, including daily routines, medical appointments, and personal care responsibilities. This detailed inventory serves as a foundation for understanding the scope of your role.

It is like creating a map; by charting out the landscape of your responsibilities, you can identify which aspects are particularly challenging. This self-awareness is crucial in managing caregiver stress, allowing you to recognize and address the most burdensome tasks and identify when outside support is warranted.

Step 2: Take Note of Your Emotions and Coping Abilities

The emotional complexity of caregiving for someone with Alzheimer's cannot be overstated. It is essential to reflect on your feelings towards this role. Do you feel overwhelmed, anxious, or resentful? Acknowledging these emotions is a vital step in understanding your coping mechanisms.

It is not uncommon for caregivers to discover that they have been underestimating the emotional toll of their duties or employing ineffective coping strategies. This realization is a key component in developing a more resilient approach to caregiving.

Step 3: Identify Sources of Support and Respite in Your Life

The next critical step is evaluating the level of support you have. This includes assistance from family members, friends, or professional services. Vigorous support can considerably alleviate the pressures of caregiving. It is important to recall that seeking help is not a sign of weakness but rather a strategic approach to maintaining your well-being and ensuring the quality of care you provide.

Step 4: Screen for Signs of Caregiver Stress

Vigilance against the signs of caregiver stress is essential. These signs can manifest as physical exhaustion, anxiety, irritability, or depression. Despite their prevalence among caregivers, these symptoms are often overlooked. Recognizing and addressing these signs early is crucial in preventing burnout and maintaining health.

If you experience multiple stress symptoms, it is advisable to consult a healthcare professional. It is no different than a gardener tending to a plant's first signs of distress, as early intervention can prevent more significant problems. So, self-awareness and appropriate action are vital to maintaining the caregiver's emotional health and building resilience.

Step 5: Re-evaluate Stressors Periodically

The nature of caregiving is such that it evolves, particularly as the person with Alzheimer's progresses in their disease. It is essential, therefore, to regularly reassess your stress factors, ideally every six months. This regular re-evaluation is like recalibrating your compass on a long journey. It permits you to adjust to changing situations, seek additional support, or access new resources. This ongoing process of assessment and adaptation is critical to managing the dynamic and often unpredictable path of caregiving.

Remember, while the caregiving journey is challenging, it is also a path of profound compassion and strength. By taking these steps, you can provide better care and safeguard your well-being.

A **worksheet** to help manage and evaluate caregiver tasks is available for your use here:

https://docs.google.com/document/d/1Pwi_XCpsoHcJP2XJ4tye
QRcDns4kQpPP/edit?usp=sharing&ouid=
106926592297134554494&rtpof=true&sd=true

From Stress to Strength: Caregivers' Strategies for Building Emotional Resilience

Emotional resilience is just like a muscle that can be strengthened over time. It is the ability to adapt and flourish despite life's challenges, and it is a skill that can be upgraded with patience and practice (Suzuki, 2021). Here, we will delve into various strategies that collectively contribute to building this resilience, insights from (Managing Stress and Building Resilience - Tips, 2022), (the National Gaucher Foundation, 2020), and (Moore, 2016). These strategies are essential in enhancing our understanding of coping with stress, overcoming adversity, and maintaining mental well-being, enabling us to navigate life's fluctuations with grace and steadiness.

1. Accept and Learn from Setbacks

How can we adapt and find constructive solutions to challenges?

Consider setbacks as stepping stones rather than stumbling blocks. Building emotional resilience involves recognizing that setbacks are a natural part of life's journey. It is about facing these challenges head-on, understanding their nature, and using them as opportunities for growth and learning. This approach involves acknowledging the difficulty of a situation while fostering a belief in one's ability to recover and advance.

2. Adopt an Optimistic Mindset

How can we shift our focus to solutions and maintain hope in challenging times?

The power of optimism in building resilience cannot be overstated. The optimistic approach is not about ignoring life's stressors but maintaining a hopeful outlook and focusing on solutions. Optimists view setbacks as temporary and within their power to overcome. This positive outlook is a catalyst for expecting good things and persisting in adversity.

3. Build Supportive Relationships

How can we strengthen connections to build a resilient support network?

The role of supportive relationships in the development of emotional resilience is critical. These relationships, whether with family, friends, or colleagues, act as a buffer against stress. They provide emotional support, practical assistance, and a sense of belonging. Cultivating these relationships involves open communication, empathy, and mutual support.

4. Practice Healthy Coping Strategies

How can we integrate coping practices into our daily routine to enhance our emotional balance and resilience?

Effective stress management and resilience building require healthy coping strategies. These include mindfulness, which anchors us in the present and reduces stress; regular physical activity, which alleviates symptoms of anxiety and depression; adequate sleep; and a balanced diet.

5. Foster Personal Meaning and Purpose

What activities or goals give a sense of purpose, and how can they guide us during challenging periods?

Discovering and pursuing what gives our lives meaning and purpose is crucial to resilience. This could be through activities that align with personal values, contributing to others' well-being, or engaging in fulfilling work or hobbies. A sense of purpose gives direction and motivation, particularly in tough times, and fills our lives with a sense of worth and fulfillment.

6. Cultivate Self-Efficacy and Mastery

How can we build this mastery and confidence in our abilities to handle life's challenges?

Developing a sense of mastery and self-efficacy in various life domains enhances resilience. This involves setting realistic goals, celebrating small victories, and acquiring new skills. A healthy sense of self-efficacy empowers us to face challenges confidently, equipped with the skills and abilities to cope effectively.

The journey to building emotional resilience is a multifaceted and proactive approach. It includes embracing a positive approach to life's challenges, learning from setbacks, maintaining optimism, nurturing supportive relationships, engaging in healthy coping strategies, finding personal meaning, and cultivating a sense of self-efficacy and mastery. These strategies, when combined, significantly enhance an individual's capacity to withstand and grow from the difficulties life presents. By adopting these practices, caregivers and individuals alike can face the complexities of life with resilience, strength, and a renewed sense of purpose.

Wrapping up this chapter, we have seen the real challenges of dementia caregiving and the incredible opportunity for personal growth. Feeling alone, anxious, or overwhelmed in this journey is normal. These emotions stem from the demanding nature of caring for a loved one whose mental abilities are declining, and it is essential to recognize how this can impact your health.

However, there is a silver lining. You have the power to become more emotionally resilient. This chapter has offered insights into understanding and managing difficult emotions, seeking support, and adopting healthy coping strategies. Embrace these tools to find personal meaning in your caregiving role and view each challenge as a chance to grow stronger.

By building emotional resilience, you are improving your well-being and enhancing the care you provide. So, take this crucial step today. Transform the stress into strength and make your caregiving journey a more positive and fulfilling experience. Remember, your emotional strength is critical in providing the best care for your loved one with dementia.

We now transition from the emotional and physical impact of dementia caregiving to the legal and practical concerns. We will equip you to navigate the complex legal issues that often arise with caregiving.

6

Legal Literacy for Caregivers

Empowerment through Understanding Rights and Obligations

Welcome, caregiving champions, to this chapter tailored to address the practical questions that often linger in your caregiving journey. This section of the book clarifies legal aspects that may weigh on your mind. Have you considered the rights and responsibilities accompanying your role as a caregiver? This chapter serves as a guide to navigating the legal dimensions of caregiving.

The legal aspects of dementia care can resemble a puzzle, sometimes leaving you uncertain and overwhelmed. Have you experienced these sentiments? If so, you are not alone. We will unravel the complexities together, providing a roadmap to address these challenges confidently. Consider those moments of anxiety regarding estate planning and power of attorney for your loved one. Have you ever wished for guidance to alleviate these concerns? This chapter addresses these common anxieties, offering insights to assuage your worries and ensure you are well-informed in your decision-making.

In Chapter 6, we are about to embark on a journey focusing on the "E" in the C.A.R.E.S.S. Method, Empowerment. Our center of the discussion is legal literacy, Part 1 of this game-changing step. This chapter is your compass, guiding you through the complexities and empowering you with the keys to confident decision-making.

Understanding Legal Literacy

As a caregiver for someone with dementia, it is critical to understand the legal aspects of caregiving. The (Legal Documents, 2024) includes essential legal and financial documents like a will, a living trust, and advance directives to ensure that a person's health care and economic decisions are carried out. It is recommended that people who have been diagnosed with some illness, such as Alzheimer's disease or related dementia, review and update their financial and healthcare plans as soon as possible. This is because the individual may lack or gradually lose the ability to make clear decisions.

Roles of Legal Literacy

Understanding the legal aspects of caring for someone with dementia might seem daunting, but it is a journey filled with respect, love, and foresight (The Importance of Legal Literacy, 2021). Imagine it as preparing a roadmap for an uncertain journey; it is about ensuring comfort and safety and honoring the traveler's wishes, who, in this case, is the person with dementia.

When someone has dementia, their ability to make decisions gradually fades away. But, like all of us, they have hopes, preferences, and desires about their care and life. By setting up legal documents early, you are giving a microphone to their voice.

Imagine a scenario where your loved one cannot express their needs or wishes. Without legal preparations like a power of attorney for health care, it is like being in a thick fog without a compass. Legal planning clears this fog. It allows a trusted replacement for themselves who can step in and navigate these decisions (The Importance of Legal Literacy, 2021).

The journey of dementia is challenging, but with early legal planning, it becomes a path paved with dignity and respect for the individual. You are not just planning; you are cherishing their wishes and ensuring their voice guides the way, even in silence. This process is a beautiful testament to the value and respect we hold for our loved ones, ensuring that their journey through dementia is handled with the care and love they deserve.

Legal Planning

Legal planning is a crucial step for individuals diagnosed with dementia and their families. It involves making important decisions and preparing documents to guide care and decision-making as the disease progresses (Legal Plans, 2019). Here are the key components of legal planning for someone with dementia:

1. Preparing for the Road Ahead

This involves deciding the type of care needed and preferred in the future. Just like packing the right clothes and essentials for a trip, legal planning includes preparing for future healthcare and long-term care needs. It is making sure that, as dementia progresses, the right kind of care is available, be it at home, in an assisted living facility, or in a nursing home.

2. Arrangements for Finances and Properties

Dementia can affect a person's ability to manage their finances. In this case, legal planning includes setting up mechanisms to manage the person's financial affairs. Suppose you plan a trip; you ensure that your home and valuables are safe. Similarly, legal planning involves taking care of finances and properties. It is like giving a trusted friend the keys to your house while you are away.

3. Choosing the Right Co-Pilot

As dementia progresses, individuals may lose the capacity to make informed decisions about their care and finances. Just as you would choose a reliable person to look after your home or pet while you are away, legal planning for dementia includes choosing someone to make decisions when the person with dementia cannot. Think of it as appointing a co-pilot who knows the route well and can keep the journey on track.

In this chapter, we will journey through the essential legal matters for those affected by dementia in an easy-to-understand and heartfelt way. Consider it as holding a guiding light and navigating the rights of patients and caregivers, ensuring their voices and choices are always heard and respected. We will then uncover the map of legal documents, from the Power of Attorney to Wills and Trusts.

Rights of Dementia Patients: Advocating for Your Loved Ones

1. Legal Capacity

Legal capacity is "the capability and power under the law of a person to occupy a particular status or relationship with another or to engage in a particular undertaking or transaction" (Merriam-Webster Dictionary, 2024). It is a fundamental human right to ensure equal treatment under the law (What Is Legal Capacity? - Legal Capacity Research, 2017).

Assessing legal capacity becomes delicate in the context of dementia. As the disease progresses, a person's mental capacity might decline, affecting their ability to understand the implications of legal documents. However, in the early stages of dementia, many individuals retain sufficient mental capacity to understand the meaning and importance of legal documents, thereby possessing the legal capacity to execute them.

2. Legal Protections

Legal protections for people with dementia are essential for safeguarding their rights and well-being. A critical aspect of legal planning for someone with dementia, drawn from Legal Rights and Protection of People with Dementia (2024), highlights the importance of not unnecessarily restricting a person's legal capacity. For instance, if an individual with dementia needs assistance in managing financial affairs, it does not automatically mean they should lose other legal rights, such as voting or making a will.

Early planning is vital for a person diagnosed with dementia. It allows the individual to express their wishes for future care and decision-making. Legal planning should cover long-term care and health care needs, arrangements for capital and property, and selecting another person to make choices on behalf of the person with dementia. This proactive approach eliminates the guesswork for families and ensures the person with dementia can designate decision-makers on their behalf (Planning Ahead for Legal Matters, 2024).

Power of Attorney (POA)

The Power of Attorney (POA) is a fundamental legal document for individuals with dementia. It empowers a person with dementia, known as the 'principal,' to designate a trusted individual, called the 'agent' or 'attorney-in-fact,' to make decisions on their behalf when they can no longer do so. This provision is essential as dementia can progressively impair the individual's ability to manage personal affairs. The agent, typically a spouse, family member, or close friend, is bestowed with the responsibility to handle financial, healthcare, and other personal matters. This role demands deep trust from the principal, as the agent must understand the significant responsibilities they are undertaking (Legal Documents, 2024).

Recognizing that the POA does not override the principal's decision-making authority if they retain legal capacity is vital. Only when the principal is deemed legally incapable does the agent assume full responsibility for managing their affairs, guided by the principal's best interests and prior wishes (Anna et al., 2021)?

1. Requirements for Signing POA

One of the primary limitations relates to the signing requirements. The person granting the POA, the principal, must have the mental capability to understand the document's consequences when signing. This means they need to comprehend the extent of the authority they give to the agent and the consequences of such delegation.

2. Finance

Regarding financial decisions, a POA typically grants the agent authority to handle the principal's financial matters. However, this authority can be limited. For instance, unless explicitly stated, the agent may not have the power to make significant decisions like selling property, altering wills, or making large financial gifts.

3. Healthcare

A healthcare POA gives the agent the authority to make medical decisions when incapacitated on the principal's behalf. However, the agent's decision-making power is often limited to what the principal has consented to in the POA document. The agent cannot make choices that go against the principal's wishes or are outside the scope of authority granted in the document.

4. General Areas

For general areas, a POA typically does not grant blanket authority to the agent in all aspects of the principal's life. There are often restrictions in place; for example, the agent may not be able to change the principal's existing will, vote in elections on behalf of the principal, or make decisions about the principal's relationships. These limitations are in place to safeguard the principal's autonomy and ensure their fundamental rights are not overridden.

Types of Power of Attorney

Understanding the types of POA can be essential in many life situations, particularly when caring for a loved one with dementia. To help you grasp the unique characteristics and applications of different types, let us explore them in detail, derived from Moric (2020).

1. Durable Power of Attorney

This type of POA remains effective even if the person granting the authority becomes incapacitated. It is beneficial in situations where ongoing decision-making power is necessary, regardless of the principal's health or mental state. Imagine a scenario where someone like Emma, who has early signs of dementia, assigns a Durable POA to her son. This enables him to manage her affairs consistently, even as her condition progresses.

2. Non-Durable Power of Attorney

Non-durable POA is designed explicitly for short-term situations and is considered invalid if the principal becomes incapacitated or dies. It is often used for specific transactions or limited periods. For instance, if Sarah travels abroad for a few months, she might grant her a Non-Durable POA to her sister to handle her financial affairs during her absence.

3. General Power of Attorney

This type grants powers to the agent, covering a wide range of personal, financial, and business matters. It is effective immediately upon signing but ceases if the principal becomes incapacitated or dies. Consider Mark, who grants a General POA to his partner before embarking on an extended overseas trip, allowing her to manage all his financial and legal matters back home.

4. Limited or Special Power of Attorney

As the name suggests, this POA is confined to specific tasks or a set timeframe. Its scope is narrowly tailored, such as authorizing someone to sell property or manage certain financial transactions. Jane, for example, might use a Limited POA to authorize her friend to sell her car while she is recovering from surgery.

5. Medical Power of Attorney

This POA type is focused on healthcare decisions. It becomes effective when the principal cannot make their own medical decisions. It is a vital tool for people who can no longer communicate their healthcare preferences due to illness or incapacity. Someone like Alex, who might face medical issues that render him unable to make decisions, could assign a Medical POA to a trusted family member or a close friend.

6. Springing Power of Attorney

Unique for its conditional activation, a Springing POA only occurs upon a specific event, typically the principal's incapacitation. This type of POA offers a sense of control and security, as it lies dormant until certain conditions are met. Jack, for example, could have a Springing POA that only activates if he is declared incapacitated by a doctor.

In cases involving a loved one with dementia, a Durable POA is often recommended. This ensures that financial, legal, and healthcare decisions can still be managed effectively as the condition progresses, maintaining a continuity of care and decision-making. Sometimes, a combination of Durable and Medical POA is recommended. They ensure that financial and healthcare decisions can be made if the individual cannot do so.

Guide Questions for Choosing a POA

These points will help you choose the most suitable POA for your loved one, providing peace of mind and the best care.

- What are the specific needs of my loved one (e.g., financial management, healthcare decisions)?
- How advanced is their condition, and how might it progress?
- Who is the most appropriate and trustworthy person to act as the agent?
- Do I need an immediate POA or one that activates under certain conditions?
- What legal processes are involved in setting up and executing a POA in my area?

When to Draft a POA?

Drafting a POA during the early stages of dementia is crucial. This timing is vital because it is at this point that the individual can still actively participate in the decision-making process. They can express their wishes regarding who will manage their affairs and how they should be managed when they can no longer do so themselves.

Why is Power of Attorney Important?

Drafting a POA during the early stages of dementia is an act of foresight and care. It ensures that the individual's preferences are respected and well taken care of when they can no longer manage their affairs.

The importance of a POA for someone with dementia cannot be overstated. It covers several critical areas:

1. Decision-making

As dementia progresses, the ability to make decisions diminishes. A POA allows a designated agent to step in, ensuring decisions are made in the best interest of the person with dementia. For example, they might choose the most beneficial social activities or therapies.

2. Financial Management

Managing finances becomes increasingly challenging. With a POA, an agent can take over tasks like paying bills, managing investments, and ensuring the individual's financial obligations are met, thus maintaining financial stability.

3. Healthcare Decisions

This includes making choices about medical treatments and living arrangements. A healthcare POA can be the difference between receiving care that aligns with the person's wishes and care that does not.

4. Legal Actions

Handling legal matters becomes complex. A POA empowers the agent to manage legal affairs such as signing contracts or filing taxes, ensuring these essential tasks are not neglected.

5. Personal Welfare

Decisions about living situations and personal care can be sensitive. The agent under a POA can decide where the person with dementia will live (at home, with family, or in a care facility) and what type of daily care they receive, aiming to maximize their comfort and well-being.

6. Deciding Successor Agents

This is about planning ahead. If the primary agent can no longer serve, the POA can specify who takes over, ensuring continuity in care and decision-making.

Who is the Agent or Attorney-in-fact?

In the context of a POA, the Agent or Attorney-in-Fact is a person appointed to act on behalf of another person, the principal. This role carries significant responsibilities and legal obligations. Let us delve into the critical roles of an Agent or Attorney-in-Fact:

1. Act According to the Principal's Wishes and in Their Best Interest

The agent's foremost duty is to act according to the principal's wishes and best interests. This means making decisions that align with the principal's wishes to the best of the agent's knowledge. If the principal's wishes are unknown, the agent must make choices based on what they believe to be in the principal's best interest. This role requires integrity and a deep understanding of the principal's values and preferences.

2. Make Financial and Other Decisions on Behalf of the Principal

The agent is often responsible for a range of decisions on behalf of the principal. This can include daily financial decisions, investment choices, and more extensive financial planning. The agent might pay bills, manage bank accounts, or even decide on buying or selling properties.

3. Manage the Principal's Income and Assets

This involves ensuring that the principal's assets are used effectively and safeguarded. The agent could handle tasks like collecting rent from properties, overseeing investment portfolios, or guaranteeing that pensions and other income sources are appropriately managed.

4. Make Healthcare Decisions for the Principal

If the POA includes healthcare decisions, the agent is responsible for medical decisions for the principal when they cannot do so themselves. This could range from choosing healthcare providers and treatments to making end-of-life care decisions. In these decisions, the agent must consider the principal's health needs, personal wishes, and quality of life.

5. Undertake Legal Actions on Behalf of the Principal

This can include signing contracts, filing taxes, or representing the principal in legal proceedings. The agent must understand the legal implications of their actions and ensure that they act within their authority's scope and in the principal's best interest.

The Agent or Attorney-in-Fact is a position of trust and responsibility. It requires a commitment to acting in the principal's best interest, making informed decisions, and managing various tasks, from financial and legal matters to healthcare decisions. The role demands integrity, competence, and a deep respect for the principal's wishes and well-being.

Wills, Living Wills, and Trusts

1. Wills

A Will is a legal document that is considered effective after death. It outlines how you want your assets distributed and can name guardians for minor children (Ramirez, 2023). A Will is crucial for individuals with dementia, as it allows them to designate how their assets should be distributed after passing. This is particularly important for ensuring their wishes are respected when they can no longer communicate them. It is advisable to create or update a will soon after a dementia diagnosis so the individual can still make informed decisions.

2. Living Wills

A Living Will takes effect if you become incapacitated and unable to make healthcare decisions. It enables individuals to express their healthcare preferences, especially in the later stages of dementia when they might be unable to make decisions themselves. This document can specify treatment preferences, life-sustaining measures, and end-of-life care, ensuring that the individual's wishes are followed even when they cannot communicate them.

3. Trusts

By setting up a Trust, persons with dementia can ensure their assets are managed as per their wishes, both during their lifetime and after their passing (Hicks, 2020). This is especially beneficial as the disease progresses, and they may no longer be able to manage their affairs.

Aspect	Wills	Living Wills	Trusts
Effectiveness Timeline	Effective upon death Guiding asset distribution after probate.	Effective upon incapacitation Guiding healthcare decisions.	Effective upon creation and asset transfer, Managing assets during and after a lifetime, often without probate.
Purpose and Function	Primarily for asset distribution after death.	Focus on healthcare preferences in case of incapacitation.	Asset management and distribution, Offering more control and privacy.
Probate and Privacy	Usually requires probate A public process.	Not related to probate They are about healthcare decisions.	Often avoids probate Providing a more private way to handle estate matters.

Table 5.1: Key Differences among the legal documents

Wills and Living Wills are essential for stating your wishes regarding asset distribution and healthcare decisions. Trusts offer a more comprehensive and private solution for managing your assets, both during your lifetime and after your death.

Importance of Wills and Living Wills

1. **Expresses Medical Wishes**: A Living Will allows individuals to specify their medical care preferences in advance, particularly when they cannot make such decisions due to dementia or terminal illness.

2. **Guides Healthcare Providers:** It provides clear instructions about the types of life-sustaining treatments or interventions an individual consents to or refuses, such as artificial life support, ensuring that medical professionals understand and respect their wishes.

3. **Legal Authority for Medical Decisions:** When individuals cannot make decisions themselves, a Living Will is a legal document that guides family members and healthcare providers in making informed decisions that align with their preferences.

4. **Avoids Family Conflicts:** By clearly stating healthcare preferences, a Living Will can prevent disputes among family members about medical decisions, reducing stress during difficult times.

5. **Reflects Personal Values and Beliefs:** It allows individuals to incorporate their values, religious beliefs, and ethical views on end-of-life care into their medical planning.

6. **Provides Peace of Mind:** Knowing that their wishes will be respected, individuals can have peace of mind about their future healthcare.

7. **Facilitates Advance Discussions:** Encourages individuals to have meaningful conversations with family members and healthcare providers about their end-of-life care preferences.

8. **Complements Other Legal Documents:** Works in conjunction with other documents like a durable POA for health care to provide a thorough approach to end-of-life planning.

9. **Customizable to State Laws:** Living Wills can be tailored to meet specific state law requirements, ensuring legal validity and effectiveness.

Importance of Trusts

1. **Name Guardians for Minor Children:** Trusts can be used to appoint guardians for children, ensuring they are cared for according to the trustor's wishes.
2. **Asset Management and Distribution:** They allow for the distribution and management of assets during the trustor's lifetime and after their death, often bypassing the probate process.
3. **Avoids Probate and Maintains Privacy:** Trusts can avoid the lengthy and public probate process, providing privacy and efficiency in handling estate matters.
4. **Flexible Control Over Assets:** Trusts offer greater control over when and how assets are distributed to beneficiaries.
5. **Can Include Specific Conditions:** Trustors can set conditions on asset distribution, such as age or milestones, providing a structured way to manage the inheritance.

- **A General Piece of Advice**

Readers should check their local laws and consult an attorney to ensure their Living Will or Trust is appropriately executed. This is crucial as laws and requirements vary significantly by state, and an attorney can provide personalized advice based on a reader's unique situation and goals.

- **How to Decide Between Will and Trust?**

When deciding between a will and a trust for someone with dementia, consider these factors, as outlined by (Ramirez, 2023). The following table provides a clear and concise comparison of wills and trusts, helping those caring for someone with dementia make an informed decision that is best suitable to their specific needs and circumstances:

Factor	Will	Trust
Cost	$0 to $1,000 (Varies with complexity)	$160 to $600+ (Simple to complex trusts)
Dependents	Ideal for naming guardians for minors	Does not cover guardianship
Process	Straightforward, less paperwork	More complex, more paperwork is required
Effect	Effective after death, includes guardianship	Effective upon signing, no guardianship
Taxes	Does not avoid estate taxes	Possible tax benefits with irrevocable trusts
Privacy	Subject to public probate	Bypasses probate, more private
Protection During Incapacity	No protection during incapacity	Offers protection if incapacitated

Table 5.2: Differences between Will and Trust

- **Is it possible to have both a will and a living trust?**

Absolutely. A living trust manages and distributes your assets during your lifetime and after, while a will enables you to name guardians for your children, choose an executor, and express your final wishes. Incorporating both a will and a trust is often recommended for a thorough estate plan (Hancock, 2024).

Guardianship

Guardianship is a crucial legal mechanism often used in situations where individuals, particularly those with dementia, are unable to make informed decisions about their care and property. In such cases, a court appoints a guardian or conservator to assume the responsibilities (Legal Documents, 2024).

The duration of guardianship in dementia cases can vary significantly. It often remains in place for as long as the individual requires decision-making assistance, which, in the context of progressive conditions like dementia, could mean several years.

Termination of guardianship occurs under specific circumstances, such as improving the individual's condition, which might be rare in progressive conditions like dementia. More commonly, the guardianship would end with the individual's passing.

Types of Guardianship

Understanding the types of guardianship is essential, especially when considering the care of vulnerable individuals, such as those with severe disabilities or older adults with cognitive impairments (National Guardianship Association, 2023). Let us explore these types in detail described by (Purpose and Types of Guardianship, 2024):

1. Guardianship over the Person

Guardianship over the person is like stepping into someone's shoes to make personal decisions for them. Imagine a scenario where an elderly relative with advanced dementia can no longer decide where to live, what medical treatments to receive, or even what to eat. In this case, a guardian over the person would make these life decisions.

This type of guardianship focuses on non-financial decisions. It includes choices about health care, living arrangements, and even social activities. The guardian's role is to ensure the individual's day-to-day life is managed in their best interests.

2. Guardianship over the Estate

Guardianship over the estate is all about managing finances and property. Consider a young adult with a significant developmental disability who inherits a large sum of money. They might not have the capability to manage this estate effectively. A guardian over the estate would handle financial transactions, invest money wisely, and ensure that the individual's property and financial assets are well-managed.

This type of guardianship is necessary when the individual can make personal decisions but cannot handle complex financial matters. The guardian's responsibilities include paying bills, collecting debts, managing investments, and even handling real estate transactions to preserve and protect the individual's financial well-being.

3. Guardianship over the Person and Estate

Sometimes, an individual might need help in both personal and financial matters. This is where guardianship over the person and the estate comes into play. For instance, an individual with no close family might suffer from a medical condition that impairs both their cognitive functions and their ability to manage finances. In such a case, a guardian would be responsible for personal and financial decisions.

This comprehensive form of guardianship combines the responsibilities of the first two types. The guardian is tasked with overseeing all aspects of the individual's life. The role requires specific skills – empathy and care in making personal life decisions and understanding and diligence in financial management.

The type of guardianship chosen depends on the specific needs of the individual in question. Whether it is making personal decisions, managing financial affairs, or a combination of both, guardianship plays a vital role in protecting and supporting those who cannot fully support themselves.

When is Guardianship Needed?

Guardianship becomes particularly important in situations where a person, often suffering from conditions like dementia, can no longer self-manage their care. Assume a scenario where an older woman, Mrs. Johnson, is diagnosed with advanced Alzheimer's disease. She struggles with daily tasks and decision-making, and there is disagreement among her family members about her care. This is a typical situation where guardianship becomes necessary.

What are the Roles of a Guardian?

In the journey of guardianship, a guardian assumes various critical roles, each playing a pivotal part in ensuring the well-being and rights of the person under their care. Let us explore these roles.

1. Determine and Monitor Residence:

The guardian decides where the person will live. This could mean choosing between home care, assisted living, or a nursing facility. Imagine being responsible for determining whether Mr. Smith, who has severe mobility issues, should stay in his two-story home or move to an assisted living facility.

2. Consent to and Monitor Medical Treatment:

Guardians consent to medical treatments and monitor their effectiveness. For instance, if Mrs. Allen needs surgery under guardianship, the guardian must understand the risks and benefits and make an informed decision.

3. Consent and Monitor Non-Medical Services:

This involves approving services like education or counseling. If a young ward, like 16-year-old Emily, needs therapy or special education, the guardian evaluates these needs and consents to the appropriate services.

4. Consent and Release of Confidential Information:

Guardians have the authority to access and permit the release of confidential information. For example, the guardian must approve if Mr. Gomez's social worker needs access to his medical records.

5. Make End-of-Life Decisions:

One of the most solemn duties involves deciding on life-sustaining treatment and other end-of-life care. If Mrs. Patel, who is terminally ill, has a guardian, this person will need to consider her beliefs and wishes when making these tough decisions.

6. Possess a Driver's License:

In some cases, guardians might be responsible for decisions about the ward's driving privileges, including whether they should retain a driver's license. This is crucial for ensuring the safety of individuals like Mr. Thompson, who has vision problems but insists on driving.

7. Act as Representative Payee:

Guardians often manage government benefits like Social Security, ensuring these funds are used for the ward's benefit. Imagine managing Mr. Lee's Social Security benefits to cover his living and medical expenses.

8. Manage, Buy, or Sell Property:

This includes handling real estate transactions and managing property. If Mrs. Rodriguez, under guardianship, inherits a property, the guardian might decide whether to keep, sell, or rent it.

9. Contract:

Guardians can enter into contracts on behalf of the person under guardianship. For example, if young Lucas needs a tutor, his guardian arranges and signs the tutoring contract.

10. File Lawsuits:

Guardians may need to file or defend lawsuits on behalf of their wards. If Ms. Johnson is wrongly denied insurance coverage, her guardian might need to pursue legal action.

Each of these roles carries immense responsibility, shaping the life and welfare of the person under guardianship.

Pros and Cons of Guardianship

When considering guardianship, it is important to weigh its advantages and disadvantages. Guardianship for a person with dementia offers numerous benefits regarding legal rights, improved quality of life, and social advantages. It also comes with responsibilities and potential complexities.

Let us discuss the pros first:

1. **Protection and Advocacy:** Guardianship ensures that the individual's interests are protected, particularly in health care and financial matters.
2. **Legal Authority:** The guardian has the legal right to make decisions, which is crucial when medical or financial decisions are necessary.
3. **Continuity of Care:** A guardian can provide a consistent approach to the individual's care, essential for those with dementia.

The cons of guardianship are as follows:

1. **Unknown Time Commitment:** The duration of guardianship can be uncertain. It could potentially last many years and require a long-term commitment from the guardian.
2. **Responsibility and Stress:** The role of a guardian comes with significant responsibilities and can be emotionally and physically taxing.
3. **Legal Complications:** Becoming a guardian involves legal proceedings, which can be complex and time-consuming.

Alternatives to Guardianship

In addressing alternatives to guardianship, particularly for individuals with dementia, it is essential to consider options that respect their autonomy while ensuring their safety and well-being. Here are some notable alternatives derived from (Supported Decision Making - Penn Memory Center, 2023) and (Clark, 2023):

1. **Representative or Substitute Payee:** This role involves managing specific financial benefits, like Social Security or Supplemental Income, on behalf of the individual. It is a more limited role than a guardian, focusing solely on finances.
2. **Case/Care Management:** This involves professionals coordinating care services and support for the individual, ensuring their needs are met without full guardianship.
3. **Health Care Surrogacy:** A healthcare surrogate makes medical decisions for the person if they cannot do so themselves. This can be a more limited and focused alternative to full guardianship.
4. **Trusts:** Establishing a trust can be a way to manage an individual's assets without needing full guardianship. Trusts can be formed in many ways to suit the individual's needs.
5. **Durable Powers of Attorney for Property:** This allows one to appoint someone to make decisions about their property and finances, and it remains effective even if the person becomes incapacitated.
6. **Durable Powers of Attorney for Healthcare:** This is similar to the above, but specifically for healthcare decisions. It ensures that a trusted person can make medical decisions if the individual cannot.

7. **Community Advocacy Systems:** These systems involve support from community resources or advocacy groups to assist individuals in making decisions or managing certain aspects of their lives.

8. **Joint Checking Accounts:** This allows a trusted person to manage banking and financial transactions, offering a simpler alternative to full financial guardianship.

9. **Community Agencies/Services:** Various community services and agencies can provide assistance and support, reducing the need for a guardian.

10. **Supported Decision-Making Networks:** This concept allows individuals with cognitive impairments to retain decision-making independence by choosing trusted friends or family members to assist in decision-making rather than having decisions made for them.

Each of these alternatives offers different levels of support and autonomy, and the best choice depends on the specific needs and circumstances of the individual with dementia.

Rights of Caregivers

As a caregiver, especially for someone with dementia, it is crucial to understand and assert your rights. This understanding helps you provide better care and ensures your well-being. Let us delve into these rights, using insights from (A Caregiver's Bill of Rights - Family Caregiver Alliance, 2014) and (Horne, 2023):

1. **Self-Care:** As a caregiver, you have the right to care for yourself. This is not selfish; it is necessary. Imagine you are on an airplane, and the oxygen masks drop down. You are instructed to put on your mask first before helping others.

This principle applies to caregiving, too. You cannot effectively care for someone if you are not well yourself.

2. **Seek Help:** It is okay to seek help from others, even if your loved one objects. Caregiving is demanding, and recognizing your limits is a sign of strength, not weakness. Think of it as assembling a team where everyone plays a vital role in providing care.

3. **Maintain Personal Life:** You have the right to maintain aspects of your life that do not include the person you are caring for. This might mean continuing hobbies, social activities, or career pursuits. Remember, caregiving is just one part of your life, not its entirety.

4. **Express Emotions:** Feeling angry, depressed, or experiencing other difficult emotions occasionally is normal. You are not a robot, and it is okay to acknowledge and express your feelings.

5. **Reject Manipulation:** If your loved one attempts to manipulate you (consciously or unconsciously) through guilt or depression, you have the right to reject this. It is essential to set boundaries to prevent emotional strain.

6. **Receive Consideration and Affection:** You deserve affection, consideration, forgiveness, and acceptance for what you do as long as you offer these qualities in return. It is a two-way street.

7. **Take Pride:** Take pride in what you are accomplishing. It often takes tremendous courage to meet the needs of a loved one with dementia. Acknowledge your efforts and the difference you are making.

8. **Protect Individuality:** You have the right to protect your individuality and make a life that will sustain you when your loved one no longer needs your full-time help. It is essential to think about your life beyond caregiving.

9. **Expect Support:** As resources for those with physical and mental impairments advance, you can expect and demand strides in support for caregivers. You are part of a larger community that deserves attention and resources.

Assessing Your Rights: To determine if you are upholding these rights, regularly reflect on your caregiving experience.

Ask yourself questions like:

- Am I taking enough time for myself?
- Am I setting boundaries for my well-being?
- Am I seeking and accepting help when needed?
- Do I feel respected and appreciated in my role?

These reflections can help you identify areas where you might need to assert your rights more firmly or seek additional support.

Remember, asserting your rights as a caregiver is not just about you. It is about providing the best possible care for your loved one by ensuring your health and happiness.

Obligations and Responsibilities of Caregivers

As a caregiver, your journey is shaped by numerous factors, including your loved one's specific needs, circumstances, and disease progression (Summerhouse Senior Living, 2023). This individualized nature of caregiving means there is no one-size-fits-all approach; instead, it requires adaptability, understanding, and patience.

In this complex role, you shoulder various obligations and responsibilities to ensure the well-being and safety of your loved one. Let us explore some key responsibilities stated by (Assisting Hands,

2021) (Understand the Dementia Caregiver's Role | Dementia Care Notes, 2010) and (5 Essential Caregiver Duties, 2019):

1. **Assistance with Daily Living Activities**: Helping with necessities such as bathing, dressing, and eating. Remember, maintaining dignity is crucial. Imagine how you would feel in their place and act accordingly.
2. **Providing Transportation**: This includes driving to medical appointments and social events. It is about physical mobility, maintaining social connections, and a sense of regularity.
3. **Establishing Routines**: Consistency can be comforting in the face of memory loss. Simple rituals, like a nightly cup of tea, can become anchors in a shifting world.
4. **Wandering Prevention**: Wandering is a common and serious concern. Strategies might include door alarms or ID bracelets. How would you feel if your loved one went missing? This fear underscores the importance of preventive measures.
5. **Safety**: Modify the living environment to minimize risks, such as installing grab bars or removing tripping hazards. Safety is as much about preventing accidents as it is about creating a secure environment.
6. **Medication Management**: Ensure medications are taken correctly and on time. It is a balancing act between respecting their independence and acknowledging their needs.
7. **Communication**: This involves adapting your communication style to their abilities. It is about listening with your heart, not just your ears.
8. **Emotional Support**: Be a source of comfort and reassurance. Remember, emotional connections can persist even as memories fade.

9. **Housekeeping**: A clean, organized space is essential for well-being. Clutter can be confusing and overwhelming for someone with dementia.

It is also imperative to establish a personal care agreement with the family. This agreement outlines your duties and sets clear expectations, helping to prevent misunderstandings and ensuring that the care provided aligns with the family's wishes and the individual's needs.

To all family caregivers, the generosity and commitment you express by taking on this all-consuming role are honored and recognized.

This chapter highlights how crucial it is for caregivers to understand the law. It is about knowing legal terms and making intelligent choices and plans. We have seen how important this is, especially for people caring for someone with dementia. Understanding legal capacity and when a person can make decisions is vital.

We also discussed essential documents like POAs, wills, and trusts. This is not just paperwork; they help caregivers make the best decisions for their loved ones. Understanding these documents means knowing when to use them and why they matter.

Finally, we focused on the caregivers knowing your loved one's rights and your own. Being a caregiver means having responsibilities, but it also means having rights that you need to know and use.

Adding these tools and knowledge about laws, rights, and documents to your caregiving toolbox will make you stronger and more confident in caring for your loved one while ensuring they are safe and well cared for.

Ensuring the long-term financial stability and security of both the caregiver and the loved one with dementia requires a dedicated focus. In the upcoming chapter, we dive into strategies for financial planning, navigating insurance complexities, and exploring resources to support the financial demands of caregiving.

7

Securing Finances

A Guide to Financial Empowerment for Caregivers

Are you feeling a bit lost with all the costs of caring for someone with dementia? You are not alone. Rest assured, we will make financial matters more straightforward and manageable and turn those worries into confidence.

This chapter is here to help you with these money questions. We will discuss the costs of caring for someone with dementia in an easy-to-understand way. It is not just about budgeting and numbers; we know it is about your life and your loved ones. You will find easy-to-follow advice to make your life easier and less stressful.

Before we dive into the heart of our chapter, let us spotlight the critical component: Step 4, Empowerment Part 2 - Financial Literacy, which stands as the 'E' in our C.A.R.E.S.S. Method. This step is all about arming you with the awareness and skills to navigate the financial landscape of dementia caregiving with confidence. Financial knowledge is not just about numbers and budgets but about empowering you to make informed decisions that benefit you and your loved one. By enhancing your financial literacy, we transform what can often feel like a daunting responsibility into an empowering journey.

What is Financial Empowerment for Caregivers?

Financial empowerment for caregivers refers to the knowledge, skills, and resources necessary to manage financial matters effectively for someone under their care. It is crucial, especially when caregivers are responsible for handling the financial affairs of individuals who are ill, elderly, or otherwise unable to manage their finances. Financial caregiving can include various activities, from paying bills and monitoring bank accounts to managing trusts, filing taxes, and holding a financial power of attorney (Lichtenberg, 2016). The caregiver's responsibilities include:

1. Protecting Assets and Credit

Caregivers must safeguard the assets and credit of the person they care for. This involves making informed investment decisions and being vigilant against fraud or financial abuse.

2. Seeking Proactive Legal and Financial Advice

This might involve consulting with financial planners or attorneys to ensure that all legal and financial actions are sound and in the best interest of the care recipient.

3. Paying for Formal Care Services

Another significant responsibility is planning for the cost of professional care services. There are times when care needs exceed what the caregiver can provide, so home health services become necessary, or considering assisted living or long-term nursing home care may become inevitable.

Financial empowerment can reduce the stress and anxiety linked with caregiving responsibilities. Knowing that the financial aspects are under control allows caregivers to focus more on their physical and emotional well-being. Let us dig into what you need to know and how to find the resources to provide the best care for your loved one.

Steps to Financial Freedom: Beginning Your Caregiving Financial Journey

As you prepare to take on the critical role of caregiver, let us explore the seven essential steps to start your caregiving financial journey, drawing wisdom from (Vittayarukskul, 2023) and (AARP, 2019).

Step 1: Review Current Finances

Firstly, assess the current financial landscape. Gathering comprehensive information about your loved one's assets, liabilities, savings, and other income sources is crucial. This step involves developing a clear picture of monthly expenses, insurance policies, and ongoing medical costs.

Step 2: Have Crucial Conversations with Family and Advisors

Open and honest communication is the key. Discuss with family members and seek advice from financial advisors. Addressing expectations, responsibilities, and concerns regarding your loved one's care and financial matters is important.

Step 3: Get Legal and Financial Powers in Place

Securing legal and financial authority, such as a power of attorney, is vital. This enables you to make decisions on behalf of your loved one, especially if they cannot do so themselves. Understanding and organizing important legal documents is a part of this process.

Step 4: Explore Support Programs

Investigate available government programs, community resources, and insurance benefits that can provide financial assistance. Many caregivers overlook this crucial step, yet it can offer significant support in managing the costs associated with caregiving.

Step 5: Make a Budget

Creating a budget tailored to caregiving needs is essential. This should include all expected expenses, such as medical bills, caregiving supplies, and potential modifications to living spaces.

Step 6: Plan Ahead

Anticipating future expenses and care needs is a critical aspect of financial planning. This foresight allows you to prepare for possible increases in care costs. Long-term care may become necessary as symptoms increase and abilities decrease, which can significantly impact the cost of care.

Step 7: Seek Guidance

Do not hesitate to seek guidance from financial planners or an eldercare attorney. They can provide valuable knowledge and help navigate the complexities of long-term financial planning for caregiving.

While distinct, each of these steps is interconnected and has a crucial role in the financial aspect of caregiving. Remember that the goal is to manage finances effectively and ensure that your loved ones have the best possible care without compromising financial stability.

Successful financial planning for caregivers requires a dynamic and proactive approach. By addressing financial planning, caregivers can better manage their responsibilities and ensure their economic well-being and those they care for.

How to Seek Financial Assistance for Caregivers

Financial support is vital in the caregiving journey, especially when the caregiver is a family member. Let us delve into how you can navigate this path with more ease and understanding.

1. Medicare

Hospital stays, and skilled therapy short stays in a nursing home are covered following a hospital stay. Hospice care and some home health care services are covered. However, Medicare does not cover long-term care, such as nursing homes and assisted living.

2. Check Eligibility for Medicaid Programs

If you qualify for Medicaid, your long-term care costs in nursing homes can be covered. Some states also pay for assisted living or in-home care. There are income limitations to qualify for Medicaid benefits, and each state has specific rules. There are also time limits on when assets can be transferred. There is usually a 5-year lookback period for asset transfers with Medicaid. Check with your state to understand the benefits available in your area.

Suppose you are caring for a family member at home and must give up your career. You may wonder, "How can I make this sustainable for both of us?" Here comes Medicaid's Self-Directed Services Program. Some states allow payment to family caregivers. These programs allow patients, including their families, to choose their caregivers. It is like managing your care staff. Contact your local Medicaid office to investigate this possibility. (Get Paid as a Carer for a Family Member | USAGov, 2023)

3. Enroll in Home and Community-Based Services (HCBS) Program

Assume your elderly parent prefers home to long-term care. Home and Community-Based Services (HCBS) excels here. It encourages long-term care in homes or communities rather than institutions and can help with equipment costs, medical supplies, and home health services.

4. Veterans Aid

Military veterans may qualify for financial aid. VA benefits for the veteran or spouse to help pay for senior care. Benefits may depend on length of service and other variables. Check with your local Department of Veterans Affairs office to help with this process.

Veterans who qualify for Veterans' Directed Home and Community-Based Services can use their flexible budget to hire a family member as a caregiver. Besides the VA pension, Aid and Attendance Benefits provide financial assistance (How to Become a Paid Carer, 2023). This can help pay for caregivers, including family members.

5. Long-Term Care Insurance

These plans are designed to cover long-term care services. Most plans also cover assisted living and in-home care. Some plans can also provide caregiver compensation, including family benefits. It can act as a safety net set up years ago to catch you in a pinch. However, coverage details can differ significantly, so reading the policy is essential.

6. Company-Provided Paid Leave

In today's world, where the balance between work and personal life is increasingly valued, some employers offer paid leave for employees who are also caregivers. It is like a bridge, helping you cross the challenging waters of caregiving without jeopardizing your professional life.

7. Family Support Consideration

Conversing with family members about contributing financially can provide additional support. It is a way of pooling resources, ensuring that the burden does not fall on just one person's shoulders, and recognizing that while not everyone can be a caregiver, everyone can contribute somehow.

8. Tax Credits and Deductions

Tax Credits and Deductions can be complex, so consulting a tax professional can be wise. This ensures you are not leaving any stone unturned in seeking financial relief.

9. Nonprofit Organization Assistance

Imagine having a network of support and resources at your fingertips. Organizations like the AARP and the Family Caregiver Alliance shine in this area, offering information, tools, and support. They can also provide educational materials, advocacy, and emotional support, helping caregivers navigate their challenges (AARP, 2019).

10. Respite Care Benefits: Essential Breaks for Caregivers

Respite care benefits, often included in various insurance policies, provide temporary relief for caregivers. This benefit allows caregivers to take necessary breaks, ensuring they do not suffer from burnout and can continue providing high-quality care. Medicare allows for respite days for the benefit of the caregiver. These services provide temporary relief, ensuring caregivers can recharge and maintain their well-being.

11. Hospice Services

Hospice organizations offer various services for caregivers and families, from medications and personal care products to counseling and education.

This chapter is an essential resource for those caring for someone with dementia. It recognizes the financial challenges caregivers and families face and emphasizes the importance of a long-term financial plan and understanding insurance options. It is a guide to help caregivers handle finances confidently while caring for their loved ones. It offers practical advice, from budgeting to seeking financial assistance, making the caregiver's financial journey less stressful.

In chapter 8, we will embark on the deeply personal and sensitive journey of long-term and end-of-life planning. We will guide you through the difficult yet crucial conversations and decisions that accompany planning to ensure your loved one's values and preferences are honored in their final days.

8

Crafting a Successful Future

Navigating Long-term Care Options and End-of-Life Planning

In the wise words of Senator John Hoeven, "Caring for our seniors is perhaps the greatest responsibility we have. Those who walked before us have given so much and made possible the life we all enjoy." This quote beautifully introduces this chapter, in which we will explore the essential steps in planning for the future of those with dementia. Our journey will guide us through the different long-term care options available, helping you understand each one. From in-home care that allows your loved ones to stay in a familiar environment to specialized facilities that offer extra support, we will try to find the right fit for you.

We will also talk about end-of-life planning. This is not easy, but it is a crucial part of caring. We will discuss how to have these tough conversations, make plans that respect your loved one's wishes, and handle the legal aspects. This is about ensuring your loved one's final years are as comfortable and dignified as possible.

Our goal is to empower you with knowledge, alleviate the weight of uncertainty, and light how to navigate these crucial decisions for your loved one, honoring their legacy and the life they have lived.

As we progress in this chapter, we reach Step 5: Success for the Future, the key 'S' in our C.A.R.E.S.S. Method. Our holistic approach to dementia care centers on this step, symbolizing forward-thinking and proactive planning. This section explores the complex world of long-term care and offers advice on choosing the right option for each dementia patient.

It is about facing the future with courage, knowledge, and empathy to write our loved ones' final phase with dignity and respect. In the spirit of the C.A.R.E.S.S. Method, we will explore the tools and knowledge to navigate these tricky waters and ensure that your path leads to success for both the caregiver and the cared-for in the future.

Embracing the Journey: Understanding Long-term Care Options and End-of-Life Planning for Caregivers

The importance of learning about long-term care options and end-of-life planning cannot be understated, especially as it relates to the later stages of dementia. Understanding and preparing for these needs is crucial for several reasons. Let us discuss them one by one:

1. Preparation for Future Needs

As people age, especially those with conditions like dementia, their care needs become more complex and demanding. The latter stages of dementia require more comprehensive care, which often requires long-term care facilities or intensive home care. This preparation is vital to ensure appropriate and compassionate care is available as the person's condition progresses (The Later Stage of Dementia, 2021).

2. Financial Planning

The cost of long-term care can be significant. Without proper planning, it can lead to financial strain on both the individual and their family. Families can better manage these expenses and avoid unexpected financial burdens by understanding the potential costs and exploring options like long-term care insurance (Elder Care Alliance, 2023).

3. Preserving Independence

Planning for long-term care is not just about ensuring that medical and physical needs are met. It is also about maintaining as much independence as possible. Putting a plan in place enables individuals to actively participate in shaping their future care and living arrangements. This autonomy is crucial for maintaining dignity and quality of life, especially for those with debilitating conditions like dementia.

4. Reducing the Burden on Family

Consideration of long-term care plans significantly reduces the burden on family members. Primary caregivers and family members often bear the burden of responsibility, which can be emotionally and physically overwhelming. Having a plan significantly eases this burden.

5. Ensuring Care Consistent with Preferences

By planning early, people can make clear choices about their future care. This means they can decide how they want to be looked after and what is important to them. Early planning is beneficial if there comes a time when they cannot express their wishes. It makes sure their needs and preferences are known and followed.

6. Reducing Stress for Loved Ones:

Knowing that there is a plan in place for long-term care can significantly reduce the stress and anxiety of loved ones. It provides a clear roadmap for care, which can be comforting during uncertainty and emotional strain.

7. Improving Quality of Life and Care

Long-term care planning can improve individuals' quality of life and care. Ensuring that care needs are met in a way that aligns with personal preferences allows individuals to enjoy a better quality of life even as their care needs increase.

8. Legal and Financial Considerations

Understanding and planning for the legal and financial aspects include considerations like wills, power of attorney, and the financial impact of different care options, ensuring that all legal and financial matters are in order.

Now that we understand the importance of long-term care and end-of-life planning let's look at the options.

Care Beyond Memory: Guide to Long-term Dementia Care Options

Long-term care options for individuals with dementia can be considered to meet the specific needs and stages of the condition. Here is an overview of the different units involved in long-term care for dementia:

1. Adult Day Centers and Respite Services

These centers offer daytime care for individuals with dementia, counseling, health services, nutrition and meals, personal care help, and various activities (music, art, recreation, support groups). They are beneficial as they give caregivers a break and ensure that the person with dementia is engaged in social and stimulating activities. The services offered can differ from center to center, so it is important to inquire about specific offerings (Osborne, 2022).

2. Retirement Housing

Retirement housing is suitable for those in the early stages of dementia. It allows individuals to live independently while providing limited supervision. These facilities often offer social activities, transportation, and other amenities, making them a good fit for those who can still manage their daily needs but may benefit from a communal living environment (Long-Term Care, 2024).

3. Assisted Living

This option bridges the gap between independent living and more intensive nursing home care. Assisted living facilities typically offer housing, meals, supportive services, and healthcare. It is important to verify that the facility has experience and services specifically designed for people with dementia (Long-Term Care, 2024).

4. Memory Care Units/Alzheimer's Special Care Units (SCUs)

These units are specifically designed to meet the needs of individuals with Alzheimer's and other forms of dementia. They may be part of larger residential care communities and can vary in form. These units usually offer specialized activities, trained staff, and an environment tailored to the needs of those with cognitive impairments.

5. Adult Family Homes

These are smaller residential care settings, typically located in neighborhood homes, offering personal care and services to a small number of residents. They provide a more intimate setting and often include services like personal care assistance, housekeeping, meals, and activities. It is essential to assess if these homes have the capability and experience to handle the specific needs of the person with dementia (Cleveland Clinic, 2024).

6. Specialized Dementia Care Facilities

These facilities are explicitly tailored for dementia patients and provide round-the-clock specialized care. They offer various services, including cognitive stimulation activities, medication management, and specially trained caregivers. These facilities are designed for the safety and specific needs of dementia patients, offering a higher level of specialized care than typical retirement homes or nursing homes.

It is critical to consider the individual's specific needs, stage of dementia, and personal preferences while choosing a long-term care option. Additionally, it is advised to visit potential facilities, ask about their services, staff qualifications, and experience with dementia care, and assess their safety and comfort level.

When to Consider Long-term Care for Your Loved One?

It is essential to recognize specific signs that indicate their needs may be beyond what home care can provide. Here is a more detailed look at each indicator:

1. Recent Accidents

Accidents such as falls or medical emergencies are critical indicators. They suggest the environment may no longer be safe for your loved one. Repeated accidents or increasing severity of incidents can indicate that your loved one requires a safer, more controlled environment where they can receive immediate assistance when needed (Freedom Village, 2022).

2. Progression of Chronic or Pre-existing Health Problems

Deteriorating health conditions, like heart disease or diabetes, can become more challenging to manage at home. Increased medical needs, such as the requirement for dialysis or frequent doctor's visits, are indicators that a more structured care setting, where medical support is readily available, might be necessary.

3. Withdrawal from Social Activities

If your loved one is increasingly withdrawing from social interactions, avoiding activities they used to enjoy, or showing a lack of interest in maintaining friendships, this could be a sign of depression or a decrease in cognitive abilities. Social withdrawal can accelerate cognitive decline, making it essential to consider environments where social engagement is encouraged and facilitated (Parkshore Wealth Management, 2022).

4. Increasing Medical Needs

If there is a noticeable increase in the complexity and frequency of medical care required – for instance, more medications, specialized treatments, or a need for constant medical supervision – this can be a strong indication that your loved one may benefit from long-term care, where medical support is an integral part of daily life (Signs It's time for long term Care, 2021).

5. Cognitive Decline

Significant memory issues, confusion, and difficulty in recognizing familiar places and people are significant signs of advancing dementia. Suppose your loved one often forgets important events, gets lost in previously familiar settings, or shows drastic personality changes. In that case, these are clear indicators that a more supportive and structured care setting might be required.

6. Caregiver Burnout

Considering you, as a caregiver, are experiencing chronic stress, emotional and physical exhaustion, or finding it difficult to manage other responsibilities due to caregiving demands, it is a sign that the current care arrangement might be unsustainable. Caregiver burnout affects your health and the quality of care you can provide (Member Benefits, 2018).

7. Difficulty Managing Household

Signs of neglect in maintaining the household, such as issues with cleanliness, unpaid bills, or poor personal hygiene, indicate that your loved one may struggle with daily living activities. This can stem from physical limitations, cognitive decline, or both, signaling the need for a living situation where these aspects are managed as part of their care.

It is essential to carefully consider these indicators in the context of your loved one's overall health and well-being. Each situation is unique, and the decision to move to long-term care should be made with careful consideration and consultation with healthcare professionals.

How to Choose the Right Long-term Care Option?

Choosing the right long-term care option for someone with dementia involves several critical steps:

Step 1: Assess Needs and Preferences

It is crucial to consider the individual's medical needs, personal preferences, and the stage of their dementia. Different types of care settings include retirement housing for those in the early stages of dementia, assisted living facilities, nursing homes for around-the-clock care, and Alzheimer's special care units designed specifically for dementia patients. Consider factors like the individual's ability to manage daily living activities, health status, and communication skills or behavior changes.

Step 2: Research Available Options

Look into various types of facilities discussed earlier in this chapter. Assisted living facilities provide independence and support, offering personal care assistance, medication management, and social activities. Skilled nursing facilities provide comprehensive medical care and support for those with complex medical needs (Understanding Long-Term Care Options for Seniors with Dementia, 2023).

Step 3: Consult with Healthcare Professionals

Engage with doctors, social workers, and other healthcare professionals familiar with the patient's condition. They can provide valuable insights into the type of care needed and may recommend specific facilities or care approaches.

Step 4: Visit Facilities

Visiting potential facilities is a must. Make visits at different times to observe the daily operations, the interaction between staff and residents, the cleanliness, and the overall atmosphere. Pay attention to how residents are cared for and whether the staff seems friendly and respectful (Finding Long-Term Care for a Person with Alzheimer's, 2017).

Step 5: Compare Costs and Quality

Assess the costs involved in different care options. Costs can vary depending on the level of care and the amenities offered. Also, evaluate the quality of care provided, the staff's training in dementia care, and the range of services available.

Step 6: Involve Your Loved One and Family

It is essential to involve the person with dementia in decision-making as much as possible, respecting their preferences and values. Additionally, family members should be included in discussions to ensure the facility aligns with everyone's expectations and the patient's best interests.

Creating a comprehensive care plan that includes medical needs, personal preferences, and emotional well-being is crucial. This plan should guide the care provided in the chosen facility and ensure the individual's needs are fully met.

Love in the Final Chapter: Understanding End-of-Life Planning for Dementia Patients

At the heart of every journey with dementia lies a path filled with memories and emotions, especially as one approaches the end of this journey. End-of-life planning in dementia care is a delicate and profound stage in this journey. This type of planning involves making decisions about the care and treatment the patient wants to receive (or not receive) as their condition progresses and they near the end of life (End-of-Life Planning, 2024).

The scope of this plan is comprehensive. It includes decisions about medical care, such as using life-sustaining treatments (like respirators or feeding tubes) and antibiotics for infections. Living wills and power of attorney are legal documents where individuals can express their wishes for end-of-life care. These directives should be discussed and known to healthcare providers and family members (Planning after a Dementia Diagnosis, 2022). Moreover, end-of-life planning also encompasses non-medical aspects like personal care preferences, where the individual would like to receive care (at home, in a clinic, etc.), and their spiritual or religious beliefs.

In dementia, the gradual loss of cognitive abilities means that individuals may eventually be unable to make or communicate their healthcare choices. By planning ahead, they can ensure that their care aligns with their values and preferences. This provides peace of mind for the individual and reduces the burden on family members and caregivers, who might otherwise have to make difficult decisions without knowing the person's wishes (End-of-Life Planning, 2024).

When to Initiate End-of-Life Planning?

When facing a dementia diagnosis, initiating end-of-life planning early in the disease's progression is crucial. Here is a breakdown of the critical factors to consider:

1. **Cognitive Decline**: Early discussions about end-of-life care are essential. At the same time, the individual can still express their priorities and understand the implications of their choices as cognitive abilities decline with the progression of dementia (Planning End-of-Life Care, 2022). For instance, early in the diagnosis, a patient named John preferred not to receive invasive treatments. This early decision-making helps ensure his future care aligns with his current wishes.

2. **Family Involvement**: Involving family members in the discussions ensures that everyone understands the patient's wishes. For example, Susan's family held a meeting where they discussed her values and preferences, including her desire for a natural end-of-life process without aggressive medical interventions. This meeting helped the family make united decisions when Susan could no longer communicate her wishes. This collaborative approach helped to respect and fulfill the preferences and reduced the emotional burden on family members.

3. **Disease Progression**: Understanding the unpredictable yet generally gradual decline in cognitive function due to dementia is crucial. For instance, considering that Bob has early-stage dementia, his family starts exploring options for assisted living facilities, anticipating his future need for 24-hour care based on the specific progression of the disease.

4. **Healthcare Professional Involvement**: Healthcare providers offer insights into the medical aspects of end-of-life care. For example, Mary's doctor explained to her family the stages of dementia and what type of medical care she might need in each stage, aiding them in making informed decisions about her future care.

5. **Legal and Financial Matters**: Addressing legal and financial issues ensures that the person's financial affairs are in order. Early in his diagnosis, George, with the help of a lawyer, set up a durable power of attorney and completed his advance directives. This ensured that when he could no longer make decisions, his chosen representative could manage his affairs according to his wishes.

6. **Patient's Wishes and Quality of Life**: Understanding and respecting patients' wishes, including their preferences for where they want to live, types of medical interventions, and views on quality of life, is central to end-of-life planning. For instance, Emma, diagnosed with dementia, indicated a strong desire to stay at home as long as possible. Her family used this information to arrange in-home care, honoring her wish for familiar surroundings and comfort in her later years.

End-of-life planning in the context of dementia ensures that the individual's values, preferences, and dignity are respected throughout their illness. This includes medical decisions, care location, financial and legal preparation, and the emotional and physical well-being of the individual and their family.

Some Inspirational Triumphs

The journey of dementia caregiving, while fraught with challenges, can also be one of profound fulfillment and growth, as illustrated by the (Three et al.'s... 2021) inspiring stories of Eileen and Marie. Eileen, whose husband was diagnosed with Alzheimer's, faced the daunting task of balancing her full-time job with the demands of caregiving. Despite the initial frustrations and feeling over-whelmed, she found a way to turn her situation into a success story. The time her husband spent in a care facility gave Eileen the much-needed break and clarity to make a pivotal decision – she quit her job to bring her husband home. This choice allowed them to spend priceless quality time together, transforming the care-giving experience into an opportunity to strengthen their bond and create lasting memories.

Marie's experience as a caregiver for her father, diagnosed with mid-stage Alzheimer's, is equally compelling. Faced with the need to juggle full-time work and caregiving responsibilities, Marie and her family adapted to their new roles with resilience and determi-nation. Their story is a testament to the power of family, adapt-ability, and the strength found in facing challenges together.

In another situation, Stella was the caregiver to her son John. John was battling cancer as well as early-onset dementia. Stella was in her 80s but did her best to care for John with her limited physical abilities. Her feelings of inadequacy and John's struggles with his diseases strained their relationship. John reluctantly agreed when the home health nurse suggested long-term care due to increasing skin breakdown. The nursing facility not only cared for all of

John's needs but also allowed for the mother/son relationship to reconnect and reinvigorate their loving bond.

These success stories resonate with the core messages of "Dementia Support for Caregivers and Families," showcasing that caregiving can evolve from a daunting responsibility into an enriching journey with empathy, adaptation, and a robust support system. They serve as powerful examples of how caregivers can find joy, growth, and fulfillment in their roles, even amidst the complexities of dementia.

In this chapter, we explored the vital and often challenging journey of long-term care and end-of-life planning, highlighting the importance of early planning and advocating for caregivers to embrace this journey as part of the caregiving process. Decisions regarding long-term care, whether at home, in an assisted living facility, or a nursing home, and even preferences for the location of death are crucial aspects of this planning. Navigating this sensitive process with care and thoroughness can bring a sense of peace and dignity to your loved one's final days.

By acknowledging that this stage of life can be filled with love and dignity, we provide caregivers with the knowledge and confidence needed to make informed decisions while navigating the complexities of long-term care and end-of-life planning.

As we move to our final chapter, we explore how caregivers can sustain their well-being through self-care practices and leveraging community resources to foster resilience and reduce the sense of isolation often experienced in caregiving roles. Prioritizing self-care practices and utilizing support systems of all types have a profound impact on well-being and foster more patience, more empathy and more resilience for the caregiver.

9

Self-Care and Community

Building Robust Support Networks for Sustained Caregiving

The road is often winding in the caregiving journey, and the weight one carries can be profound. Yet, amidst the complexities of caring for a loved one with dementia, there lies a fundamental truth, beautifully captured by Eda LeShan: "When we truly care for ourselves, it becomes possible to care far more profoundly about other people. The more alert and sensitive we are to our needs, the more loving and generous we can be toward others." (Inspirational Quotes for Caregivers - Freedom Care, 2020). This chapter is a testament to that very essence. It is not just a guide but a gentle reminder that nurturing your well-being is not a luxury but a necessity.

In this chapter, we dive into the heart of self-care and community support. We will learn to care for ourselves in ways that keep us strong and ready to help our loved ones. It's all about finding the right balance - taking enough time for your health and happiness so that you can be there for others. We'll share easy, effective ways to look after your well-being, helping you stay refreshed and focused.

Then, we move on to building your support network. This part is about connecting with people - family, friends, and professionals who understand what you're going through. We'll show you how to create a circle of support, a group that can offer help, advice, and a listening ear when needed.

This chapter focuses on Step 6: Self-care and Support, the crucial 'S' in our C.A.R.E.S.S. Method. It is a ray of hope and strength for caregivers and families. We emphasize how a caregiver's resilience stems from self-care and building a supportive network, underscoring the importance of self-care as an essential, not optional, part of effective caregiving. Join us in learning how to create a solid and supportive environment that empowers caregivers and their loved ones to not only endure but flourish amidst the challenges of dementia.

Caring for the Caregiver: Maintaining Your Well-being Through Self-care

Self-care is taking an active role in protecting one's well-being, particularly during periods of stress. It's about recognizing and addressing your own needs, both physically and emotionally. This could involve activities that relax and revive you, like reading, exercising, meditating, or spending time in nature. It also includes more fundamental aspects like eating a healthy diet, getting enough sleep, and seeking medical care when necessary. Self-care is not selfish; instead, it's a crucial aspect of maintaining a balance in life, especially for those who spend much of their time caring for others. It's about being as kind to yourself as you are to others, ensuring you're at your best to offer support and care to those who depend on you (Family Caregiver Alliance, 2020).

Self-care for a dementia caregiver involves a series of steps and activities that the caregiver undertakes to maintain their own health and well-being while caring for someone with dementia. This can include managing stress through relaxation techniques, seeking social support, and taking time for personal interests and hobbies (Creating a Caregiving Self-Care Plan, 2022). Engaging in self-care helps prevent burnout and ensures the caregiver can continue to be present and supportive in their caregiving role (Caring for the Caregiver: 25 Ways to Care for Yourself, 2022)

Myths of Self-Care for Dementia Caregivers

When caring for a dementia patient, addressing common misconceptions surrounding self-care is crucial. If left unchallenged, these myths can lead to unnecessary strain and compromise the quality of care provided. Let's explore and debunk some of these prevalent myths to shed light on the realities of dementia caregiving and the significance of caregiver self-care.

Myth 1: Self-care is time-consuming and needs to be planned in advance

Self-care can be integrated into everyday activities and does not necessarily require large chunks of time. Caregivers can weave self-care moments into their daily routine, like enjoying their favorite playlist while doing chores or indulging in a special body wash during a shower. These small acts, known as "mini moments" of self-care, are meaningful and can significantly contribute to a caregiver's overall well-being (Dementia Caregiver Myths, 2019).

Myth 2: I feel fine, I don't need self-care

The necessity of self-care isn't always immediately apparent, especially when a caregiver feels okay. However, self-care is crucial for maintaining long-term emotional, physical, and mental health. It is an ongoing process that helps deal with the stress and demands of caregiving. Engaging in self-care activities can prevent burnout and ensure that caregivers remain effective and compassionate in their roles (Debunking 6 Myths about Becoming a Caregiver, 2023).

Myth 3: Self-care is a luxury

Self-care is not a luxury but a vital aspect of maintaining caregivers' health and well-being. It doesn't have to be expensive or extravagant. Simple, cost-free activities like listening to music, practicing meditation, or exercising at home can be effective forms of self-care. These activities do not require extra money and can be incorporated easily into daily life.

Myth 4: Home care is inadequate for Alzheimer's and dementia patients

The misconception that only professionals can provide good care for individuals with dementia is not true. While professional care services are valuable, family members and loved ones can also provide high-quality, compassionate care with the proper education and training. Educating oneself about dementia and developing effective coping strategies are essential for providing effective home care.

Myth 5: Family members can't handle the responsibility of home care

This myth underestimates the capabilities of family caregivers. While caregiving for a person with dementia can be challenging, many family members effectively shoulder this responsibility. With the proper support and resources, family caregivers can provide compassionate and competent care, although it's important for caregivers to recognize their limits and seek help when needed (Ma, 2023).

Myth 6: Seniors in memory care communities are heavily medicated

The belief that seniors in memory care communities are heavily medicated is a misconception. While medication can be a part of the treatment plan for some individuals with dementia, it is not the sole focus. Memory care communities often emphasize personalized care plans that include a variety of therapies and activities designed to enhance the quality of life and cognitive function, not just medication management.

Myth 7: Moving to assisted living leads to boredom and loss of independence

The idea that moving to assisted living facilities leads to boredom and loss of independence is misleading. Many assisted living communities provide a range of activities, social opportunities, and individualized care that can enhance the residents' quality of life. These facilities aim to support the independence of their residents as much as possible, offering various levels of assistance based on individual needs. The focus is often on maintaining an active, engaging, and socially connected lifestyle for seniors.

These myths highlight the importance of understanding the true nature of self-care and home care in dementia caregiving. By debunking these myths, caregivers can adopt more effective and sustainable practices for their own welfare and those they care for.

How do you know when you need self-care as a dementia caregiver?

The short answer to this question is always. Self-awareness is key. Recognizing when you need self-care as a dementia caregiver is vital, and there are several signs to watch for. Feeling over-whelmed, anxious, or depressed are clear indicators that the stress of caregiving is impacting your mental health. This is often accompanied by physical and psychological exhaustion, signaling that the demands of caregiving are too much (Smith, 2018).

Many caregivers struggle to balance their responsibilities with their personal lives, leading to difficulties concentrating, sleep disturbances, and changes in eating habits or weight. These are all signs that you're not taking enough time for yourself (Dementia and Family Stress, 2021). When your life seems to revolve predominantly around caregiving, with little personal satisfaction or time for self-care, it's a sign that you need to reevaluate and find a better balance.

Increased impatience and irritability can be signs of burnout, particularly towards the person you're caring for. Similarly, feelings of hopelessness or experiencing mood swings can indicate that the stress of caregiving is taking a toll on your mental well-being. Physical symptoms, like headaches or stomachaches, should not be overlooked as they can be manifestations of the stress you're under.

It's important to ask for and accept help from family, friends, or professional caregivers to manage this stress and prevent burnout.

Setting reality-based goals and boundaries can help you manage your workload and minimize feeling overwhelmed. Prioritizing your health is crucial, which includes eating well, staying active, and getting enough sleep. Regular health check-ups are also essential for your well-being.

Mastering the Art of Self-Care: Proven Strategies for Personal Wellness

Caring for a loved one with dementia is a challenging and emotionally intense role. Caregivers must engage in self-care to maintain their health and well-being. Here are some strategies:

1. Forgive Yourself

Recognize that it's normal to feel overwhelmed or impatient at times. Caregiving is demanding, and it's important to have grace for yourself when things don't go as planned or when you react in a way you didn't intend (From a Dementia Caregiver, 2023).

2. Rethink Your Expectations

Adjust your daily expectations to align with the reality of dementia caregiving. Understand that each day can be unpredictable and that it's okay if everything is not accomplished as planned. This mindset helps manage stress and avoid feelings of failure or frustration.

Accept that the needs and abilities of your loved one with dementia will change over time. Consider new forms of support, like professional care or support groups, as part of your caregiving approach.

3. Develop Healthy Goals

Prioritize your physical well-being by maintaining a balanced diet, exercising regularly, and ensuring adequate sleep. These practices boost your overall well-being and provide the stamina needed for caregiving demands.

One practical approach is to schedule a regular physical checkup, ensuring health needs are not overlooked amidst caregiving responsibilities. This step is crucial for early detection of any health issues and for receiving professional health advice. Additionally, caregivers can plan for a half-hour break once a week, allowing them some much-needed time for relaxation or personal activities. Such breaks are vital for mental and emotional rejuvenation. Lastly, incorporating a simple exercise routine, such as walking for 10 minutes three times a week, can significantly enhance physical and mental well-being (Taking Care of You, 2023).

4. Keep an Open Mind

Embrace the evolving nature of your caregiving role. Understanding that your loved one's needs and abilities will change over time is crucial. This mindset helps you adapt to new challenges and be open to considering different forms of support, such as professional care or support groups (Ma, 2023).

5. Honor Moments of Connection

Cherish the moments of clarity and connection with your loved one. Walking together, listening to music, or dancing can create meaningful interactions. Celebrate these moments and use them as a source of strength and motivation in your caregiving journey.

6. Take Breaks

Regular breaks are essential to prevent burnout and recharge. Even small breaks can make a huge difference. Consider options like respite care, where someone else takes over caregiving duties for a period, allowing you to rest and engage in activities you enjoy (Alzheimer's Caregiving, 2017).

7. Manage Stress

Incorporate stress management techniques into your routine. This could include physical activities like walking or yoga. Joining a community sports league or a group exercise class can also be beneficial.

8. Calm Your Mind

Powerful tools like mindfulness practices or meditation can be exceptionally beneficial, as they help reduce stress and improve mental clarity. Caregivers are often recommended to set aside a few minutes each day for these practices to help center their thoughts and emotions. Engaging in relaxing activities, such as reading, gardening, or listening to soothing music, can provide a mental break from the rigors of caregiving.

9. Take Care of Your Health

Eating a balanced diet full of healthy meals and snacks provides the necessary energy and nutrients to handle the physical demands of caregiving. Prioritizing sleep is also essential, as lack of rest can lead to burnout and health complications. Regular physical activity, whether walking, yoga, or vigorous exercises, is critical for maintaining physical health and managing stress. And remember, regular check-ups are crucial for early diagnosis of any health issues arising from the physically demanding caregiving role.

10. Stay Organized

Maintaining a daily journal or planner helps track essential tasks, appointments, and medication schedules. Utilizing checklists and setting reminders can further streamline the caregiving process. In today's digital age, various apps and technological tools are available to assist caregivers in staying organized, which can significantly reduce stress and improve the quality of care provided.

11. Manage Your Emotions

Recognizing, accepting, and appropriately managing emotions is crucial for a caregiver's mental health. Feelings of frustration, grief, or joy are valid and should be acknowledged. Sharing your feelings and experiences with friends and family members who understand can provide significant emotional relief.

12. Engage in Activities You Enjoy

Indulging in enjoyable activities is a vital aspect of self-care. For instance, dancing to a favorite song from your teenage years can be an uplifting and energizing experience. This type of physical activity serves as a stress reliever and rekindles pleasant memories, boosting your mood.

Similarly, a bubble bath while reading a book or magazine offers a double benefit of relaxation and escapism. It's a perfect way to unwind and take a break from the pressures of caregiving. Flipping through a coffee table book with beautiful photographs is another serene activity. It's visually stimulating and mentally relaxing, providing a quiet moment to appreciate art and beauty.

Listening to audiobooks with headphones is another effective way to take a mental break. It allows you to immerse yourself in stories or learn new things while being engrossed in the narrative.

13. Strengthen Your Support Network

Maintaining regular contact with friends is crucial for emotional support and staying socially connected. Finding a caregiver advocate can offer guidance and resources tailored to your unique caregiving situation, providing much-needed advice and support. The National Institute of Aging, the CDC, and the National Alliance on Caregiving, or AARP, are excellent caregiver advocacy resources.

Joining a caregiver support group offers a space to share experiences, gain practical advice, and feel understood by others facing similar challenges. These gatherings can be a source of comfort and camaraderie. Facebook has many wonderful dementia support groups that are always available to join and offer a platform to share your feelings with others who understand your challenges.

Building a solid support network is essential. It provides practical help, emotional support, and a sense of community, all necessary for managing the demands of caregiving.

This insightful chapter delves into the critical yet often overlooked aspect of caregiving: self-care and the formation of robust support networks. As a caregiver, especially in the challenging context of dementia care, your well-being is paramount. The chapter discusses common myths surrounding self-care for dementia caregivers, emphasizing that self-care is not a luxury but a necessity. It then offers practical, proven strategies for maintaining personal wellness, reminding readers that caring for oneself is not selfish but essential for sustained caregiving.

Ultimately, this chapter conveys empowerment, self-compassion, and practical wisdom that resonates deeply with anyone in the caregiving role. With a loving reminder that in the caregiving journey, taking care of yourself is crucial for both you and those you care for.

Conclusion: Heart of the Matter

Core Insights from the Book

As we draw the curtain on the insightful journey through "Dementia Support for Caregivers and Families," it's essential to reflect on the profound transformation that understanding, compassion, and strategic caregiving can bring to the lives of both caregivers and those living with dementia. This book, rooted in compassionate insights, equipped us with the tools and knowledge to navigate the complex terrain of dementia care and illuminate the path toward finding joy, connection, and resilience in what may often seem like an insurmountable challenge.

The C.A.R.E.S.S. Method, alongside the "Ten Absolutes" of Alzheimer's Care, forms the backbone of a caregiving philosophy that transcends conventional approaches, advocating for a blend of empathy, patience, and practical strategies. Through the compelling narratives of Edgar, Jennette, Glenda, and many others, we've seen the embodiment of these principles in real-world caregiving scenarios, offering us a beacon of hope and a testament to the human spirit's indomitable strength.

As we venture forward, it's crucial to carry the essence of these teachings in our hearts and minds. The journey of caregiving, fraught with challenges and uncertainties, also holds moments of unparalleled beauty, deep connection, and personal growth. The book's core message encourages us to view dementia care not just as a duty but as an opportunity to deepen bonds, celebrate small victories, and foster a nurturing environment that honors the dignity and identity of our loved ones.

In embracing the strategies outlined in this book, caregivers can find solace in knowing they are not alone. The shared experiences, practical advice, and emotional support woven through the pages serve as a constant companion on this journey. By prioritizing communication, empathy, and self-care, caregivers can mitigate the stress and isolation often accompanying dementia care, paving the way for a more fulfilling caregiving experience.

Furthermore, the book's emphasis on building a support network underscores the importance of community in the caregiving journey Whether through family, friends, or support groups, the collective wisdom, strength, and compassion of a community can provide the necessary support to navigate the complexities of dementia care with grace and resilience.

Embrace the caregiving journey with the insights, examples, and guidance offered in this book. It is more than a resource; it's a companion that transforms your perspective on providing care. It's about enriching and deepening your relationship with your loved ones, turning the challenges of dementia caregiving into opportunities for growth, connection, and fulfillment. You are not alone on this journey and armed with the powerful strategies and heartfelt advice from this book, you can navigate the complexities of caregiving with confidence and compassion.

"Dementia Support for Caregivers and Families" presents a philosophy of care that champions love, understanding, and patience. It invites us to see beyond the challenges of dementia, to the heart of what it means to care for another human being in their most vulnerable moments. Let us step forward with renewed purpose, armed with the knowledge that in the act of caring for another, we discover the depth of our capacity for love, compassion, and joy. Let this book be a guide, a source of comfort, and a reminder that in the shared human experience of caregiving, there is always hope, always a reason to persevere, and always an opportunity to find joy in the journey.

Leave Your Thoughts in a Review

Will you extend a hand of support to another dementia caregiver or family member? Your words could make the difference for someone in need.

All you have to do is go scan the QR code below and be the light for another today.

Leave your review here:

My heartfelt gratitude goes out to you for the positive impact you bring to the world. It's your courage and your commitment that inspires me. Thank you for all you do.

Hanna

About the Author - Hanna Wells

Hanna's professional path led her to the long-term care sector, where she found her true calling. Her career as a nursing home administrator allowed her to combine her administrative skills with her passion for elder care. Her dedication to improving the quality of life for the elderly has been a hallmark of her career.

Recently retired, Hanna continues her journey of dedication with a legacy of compassion to inspire those around her, impacting the lives of many with this, her first book.

A Note from Hanna

Dear Readers,

I want to take a moment to express my deepest gratitude to each of you. Your decision to journey through these pages is a testament to your strength, love, and commitment to those you care for. This book was born out of a heartfelt desire to provide a beacon of hope and a guide through the dementia caregiving journey.

To the caregivers and families who have opened your hearts and homes in the face of dementia, your courage is immeasurable. Thank you for allowing me to be a part of your journey. Your experiences and feedback are invaluable to me and the countless others walking this path alongside you.

I also want to extend my appreciation to the healthcare professionals, support workers, and advocates who dedicate their lives to making a difference in the lives of those affected by dementia. Your compassion and expertise are the pillars upon which caregivers can lean.

As you continue your caregiving journey, remember, you are not alone. I invite you to reach out with your stories, questions, or insights. Your voice is a powerful tool in the collective effort to support and uplift one another. Please feel free to contact me at admin@kakupublishing.net. Your contributions can help shape the future of dementia care, offering hope where it's needed most.

Together, let's continue to build a community grounded in understanding, empathy, and unwavering support. Here's to finding the strength in the stories we share, the knowledge we gain, and the connections we foster.

With warmest regards,

Hanna, Author of "Dementia Support for Caregivers and Families"

References

10 Early Signs and Symptoms of Alzheimer's and Dementia. (2024). Alzheimer's Disease and Dementia. https://www.alz.org/alzheimers-dementia/10_signs

5 Common Misconceptions About Dementia | Alzheimer's Foundation of America. (2021, August 3). Alzheimer's Foundation of America. https://alzfdn.org/5-common-misconceptions-about-dementia/#:

5 Essential Caregiver Duties. (2019, September 18). 5 essential caregiver duties when caring for a parent with dementia - Elizz. https://www.elizz.com/planning/caregiver-duties/

5 Myths About Dementia | Pfizer. (2023). Pfizer.com. https://www.pfizer.com/news/articles/5_myths_about_dementia#:

A-Z Quotes.(n.d.) Top 25 Quotes by Leo Buscaglia. Retrieved January 20, 2024. From https;//www.azquotes.com/author/2238-Leo_Buscaglia

A Caregiver's Bill of Rights - Family Caregiver Alliance. (2014). Caregiver.org. https://www.caregiver.org/resource/caregivers-bill-rights/

AARP. (2019, December 6). Tips for First-Time Family Caregivers. AARP; AARP. https://www.aarp.org/caregiving/basics/info-2019/first-time-caregiver-tips.html

AARP. (2019, November 7). Tax Tips for Caregivers. AARP; AARP. https://www.aarp.org/caregiving/financial-legal/info-2017/tax-tips-family-caregivers.html

Allado, K. (2017). Legal Planning for Dementia Patients | SeniorCareHomes.com. Seniorcarehomes.com. https://seniorcarehomes.com/senior-living-articles/medical-conditions/legal-planning-for-dementia-patients/

Allen, K. (2021, August 16). Three Experienced Alzheimer's and Dementia Caregivers Share Their Stories and Lessons | BrightFocus Foundation. Brightfocus.org. https://www.brightfocus.org/alzheimers/article/three-experienced-alzheimers-and-dementia-caregivers-share-their-stories-and

Alzheimer's Caregiving. (2017). National Institute on Aging. https://www.nia.nih.gov/health/alzheimers-caregiving/alzheimers-caregiving-caring-yourself

Alzheimer's disease. (2023, April 13). Alzheimer's Society. https://www.alzheimers.org.uk/about-dementia/types-dementia/alzheimers-disease

Amy, A. (2010, October 30). Mom with dementia confuses daughter. Chicago Tribune. https://www.chicagotribune.com/lifestyles/ct-xpm-2010-10-30-ct-live-1030-amy-20101030-story.html

Anna Smith Haghighi. (2021). Dementia and power of attorney: What to know.

Medicalnewstoday.com. https://www.medicalnewstoday.com/articles/how-to-change-power-of-attorney-for-someone-with-dementia

Assisting Hands. (2021, April 23). What are the Responsibilities of a Dementia Caregiver? Assisting Hands Home Care - Batavia IL. https://assistinghands.com/47/illinois/batavia/blog/dementia-caregiver-duties/

Behavior & Personality Changes. (2014). Memory and Aging Center. https://memory.ucsf.edu/caregiving-support/behavior-personality-changes

Brandon, P. (2017, July 21). Empathy Training for Dementia Care – A Strong Foundation Tool |. Ageucate.com. https://www.ageucate.com/blog/?p=1013#:

Can you prioritize both caregiving and wealth-building? (2023). Corebridgefinancial.com. https://www.corebridgefinancial.com/rs/home/financial-education/education-center/money-management-basics/caregiving-and-wealth-building

Caregiver Statistics: Health, Technology, and Caregiving Resources - Family Caregiver Alliance. (2016). Caregiver.org. https://www.caregiver.org/resource/caregiver-statistics-health-technology-and-caregiving-resources/

Caregiver Stress. (2024). Alzheimer's Disease and Dementia. https://www.alz.org/help-support/caregiving/caregiver-health/caregiver-stress

Caregiver Stress. (2024). Alzheimer's Disease and Dementia. https://www.alz.org/help-support/caregiving/caregiver-health/caregiver-stress

Caregiver Support: The Importance of Seeking Help When You Need It - Institute on Aging. (2014, September 19). Institute on Aging. https://www.ioaging.org/aging/caregiver-support-importance-seeking-help-need/

Caregiver's Guide to Understanding Dementia Behaviors - Family Caregiver Alliance. (2022). Caregiver.org. https://www.caregiver.org/resource/caregivers-guide-understanding-dementia-behaviors/#ten-tips

Caregivers and life insurance: What you need to know | Voya.com. (2020). Voya.com. https://www.voya.com/blog/caregivers-and-life-insurance-what-you-need-know

Caring for the Caregiver: 25 Ways to Care for Yourself. (2022, January 13). CaringBridge. https://www.caringbridge.org/resources/care-for-the-caregiver/

Clark, A. (2023, November 9). The Senior List. The Senior List. https://www.theseniorlist.com/elder-law/guardianship/

Cleveland Clinic. (2024, January 3). Long-Term Care Options for Someone With Alzheimer's Disease. Cleveland Clinic; Cleveland Clinic. https://health.clevelandclinic.org/long-term-care-for-alzheimers-patients

Clinic, C. (2022). Dementia: Symptoms, Types, Causes, Treatment & Risk Factors. Cleveland Clinic. https://my.clevelandclinic.org/health/diseases/9170-dementia

Communicating and dementia. (2023). Alzheimer's Society. https://www.

alzheimers.org.uk/about-dementia/symptoms-and-diagnosis/symptoms/communicating-and-dementia

Communication and Alzheimer's. (2024). Alzheimer's Disease and Dementia. https://www.alz.org/help-support/caregiving/daily-care/communications

Communication challenges and helpful strategies. (2022). Alzheimer Society of Canada. https://alzheimer.ca/en/help-support/im-living-dementia/managing-changes-your-abilities/communication-challenges-helpful

Connolly, C. (2021, February 25). 10 Ways to Develop Patience as a Caregiver. Guideposts. https://guideposts.org/positive-living/health-and-wellness/caregiving/family-caregiving/advice-for-caregivers/10-ways-to-develop-patience-as-a-caregiver/#:

Dealing with the Dementia, B. (2018, February 19). Dealing with the Dementia Communication Barrier | myLifeSite. MyLifeSite. https://mylifesite.net/blog/post/dealing-dementia-communication-barrier/

DeAngelis, T. (2023). Improving the quality of life for patients with dementia and their caregivers. Https://Www.apa.org. https://www.apa.org/monitor/2023/04/continuing-education-patients-dementia-caregivers

Debunking 6 Myths About Becoming a Caregiver. (2023, May 10). Discovery Village. https://www.discoveryvillages.com/senior-living-blog/debunking-6-myths-about-becoming-a-caregiver-to-people-living-with-dementia/

Dementia - communication. (2014). Dementia - communication. Vic.gov.au. https://www.betterhealth.vic.gov.au/health/conditionsandtreatments/dementia-communication

Dementia - Symptoms and causes. (2023). Mayo Clinic; https://www.mayoclinic.org/diseases-conditions/dementia/symptoms-causes/syc-20352013

Dementia and Family Stress. (2021, December 27). ReaDementia. https://readementia.com/dementia-and-family-stress/

Dementia and language. (2023). Alzheimer's Society. https://www.alzheimers.org.uk/about-dementia/symptoms-and-diagnosis/symptoms/dementia-and-language

Dementia Caregiver Myths. (2019). Careblazers.com. https://www.careblazers.com/blog/dementia-caregiver-myths-4-caregiver-myths-stopping-you-from-living

Diane. (2020, September 28). 20 Inspirational Quotes For Caregivers. NursingHomeVolunteer.com. https://nursinghomevolunteer.com/16-inspirational-quotes-for-caregivers/

Dr. Nathan Herrmann. (2016, September 9). Everything you need to know about dementia & legal issues. Your Health Matters. https://health.sunnybrook.ca/mental-health/dementia-legal-issues/

Ducharme, J. (2018, October 25). The Hidden Reasons Why Alzheimer's

Caregivers Are So Stressed. TIME; Time. https://time.com/5434345/alzheimers-caregivers-struggle/

Elder Care Alliance. (2023, October 22). 4 Reasons Why Long-Term Care Planning Is Important - Elder Care Alliance. Elder Care Alliance. https://eldercarealliance.org/blog/long-term-care-planning-importance/

Empathy in Caregiving, in. (2023, September 28). Care Plans Now. Care Plans Now . https://www.careplansnow.com/resources/empathy-in-caregiving-why-it-matters-and-how-to-cultivate-it

End-of-Life Planning. (2024). Alzheimer's Disease and Dementia. https://www.alz.org/help-support/i-have-alz/plan-for-your-future/end_of_life_planning

Explanation of the functions of the brain. (2021, March 18). Alzheimer's Society. https://www.alzheimers.org.uk/about-dementia/symptoms-and-diagnosis/how-dementia-progresses/function-brain#content-start

Family Caregiver Alliance. (2020). Caregiver.org. https://www.caregiver.org/

Financial Planning for Caregivers | FSL.org. (2023, May 30). FSL. https://www.fsl.org/financial-planning-for-caregivers-tips-and-resources-for-long-term-care/

Financial Planning for Family Caregivers. (2023, March 28). Family Caregivers Online. https://familycaregiversonline.net/caregiver-education/financial-planning-for-family-caregivers/

Finding Long-Term Care for a Person with Alzheimer's. (2017). National Institute on Aging. https://www.nia.nih.gov/health/long-term-care/finding-long-term-care-person-alzheimers

Freedom Village. (2022, May 16). Signs Your Loved One Might Need Long-Term Care - Freedom Village. Freedom Village. https://fvhollandseniorliving.com/blog/signs-you-need-long-term-care/

From a dementia caregiver. (2023, March 15). HopeHealth; HopeHealth. https://www.hopehealthco.org/blog/from-a-dementia-caregiver-10-tips-for-self-care/

Get paid as a caregiver for a family member | USAGov. (2023). Usa.gov. https://www.usa.gov/disability-caregiver

Grewal, R. (2022). The Importance of Self-Care for Family Caregivers - UF Health Jacksonville. Ufhealthjax.org. https://ufhealthjax.org/stories/2022/the-importance-of-self-care-for-family-caregivers

Hancock, J. (2024). Will vs Revocable Living Trust? | John Hancock. JohnHancock. https://www.johnhancock.com/ideas-insights/will-vs-living-trust.html

Helena, M. (2021, August 17). 10 financial planning tips for new caregivers. Ontario Caregiver Organization. https://ontariocaregiver.ca/10-financial-planning-tips-for-new-caregivers/

Helping Caregivers. (2022, January 4). Helping Caregivers with Financial Planning. Helpr-App.com. https://resources.helpr-app.com/helping-care

givers-with-financial-planning

Heltemes, M. (2016). Patience for Alzheimer's Dementia Caregviers. Mind-Start.com. https://www.mind-start.com/Developing-Patience-for-Alzheimers-Caregiving_b_170.html#:

Hicks, P. (2020, October 15). What is the Difference Between a Will and a Trust. Trust & Will; Trust & Will. https://trustandwill.com/learn/difference-between-trust-and-will

Horne, J. (2023, September 26). A Caregiver's Bill of Rights. Caregiver.com. https://caregiver.com/articles/caregivers-bill-of-rights/

How to Become a Paid Caregiver. (2023, October 30). How to Become a Paid Caregiver for a Family Member: 6 Steps to Uncovering Financial Assistance Options for Family Caregivers. Careforth. https://careforth.com/blog/how-to-become-a-paid-caregiver-for-a-family-member-6-steps-to-uncovering-finan cial-assistance-options-for-family-caregivers/

How to communicate with a person with dementia. (2021, December 20). Alzheimer's Society. https://www.alzheimers.org.uk/about-dementia/symp toms-and-diagnosis/symptoms/how-to-communicate-dementia

Huey, J (1996). https://www.alztennessee.org/help/caregiver-support/caregiver-resource-library/10-absolutes-of-alzheimers-care

Huey, J (1996). https://www.alztennessee_org/help/caregiver-support/caregiver-resource-library/10-absolutes-of-alzheimers-care

Ten Absolutes (@Huey, 1996)

Inspirational Quotes for Caregivers - Freedom Care. (2020, May). Freedom Care. https://freedomcare.com/caregiver-quotes/

Insurance Bee Inc. (2024). Business insurance. Insurancebee.com. https://www. insurancebee.com/caregivers-insurance

Is dementia hereditary? (2023). Alzheimer's Society. https://www.alzheimers.org. uk/about-dementia/is-dementia-hereditary#:

Kerr, N. (2021, June 29). Caregivers Spend More Than $7,200 a Year on Out-of-Pocket Costs. AARP; AARP. https://www.aarp.org/caregiving/financial-legal/info-2021/high-out-of-pocket-costs.html

Legal Documents. (2024). Alzheimer's Disease and Dementia. https://www.alz. org/help-support/caregiving/financial-legal-planning/legal-documents

Legal Documents. (2024). Alzheimer's Disease and Dementia. https://www.alz. org/help-support/caregiving/financial-legal-planning/legal-documents

Legal Plan. (2019). from https://alz.org/media/documents/alzheimers-dementia-legal-plans-b.pdf

Legal Planning. (2024). Alzheimer's Disease and Dementia. https://www.alz.org/help-support/i-have-alz/plan-for-your-future/legal_planning

Legal rights and protection of people with dementia. (2024). Alzheimer Europe.

https://www.alzheimer-europe.org/policy/positions/legal-rights-and-protection-people-dementia

Lichtenberg, P. (2016). Financial Empowerment for Family Caregivers Overview Older Adult Nest Egg and Successful Aging through Financial Empowerment (SAFE). https://iog.wayne.edu/events/peter_lichtenberg_presentation.pdf

Long-Term Care. (2024). Alzheimer's Disease and Dementia. https://www.alz.org/help-support/caregiving/care-options/long-term-care

Ma, T. (2023, December 12). Self-Care Strategies for Dementia Caregivers. Sagecare. https://www.sagecare.ca/blog/self-care-strategies-for-dementia-caregivers

Managing stress and building resilience - tips. (2022). Mind.org.uk. https://www.mind.org.uk/information-support/types-of-mental-health-problems/stress/managing-stress-and-building-resilience/

Member Benefits. (2018, March 22). How To Know When A Loved One Needs Long-Term Care. Member Benefits. https://memberbenefits.com/how-to-know-when-a-loved-one-needs-long-term-care/

Merriam-Webster Dictionary. (2024). Merriam-Webster.com. https://www.merriam-webster.com/dictionary/legal%20capacity

Moore, M. (2016, May 17). Mindfulness: The Art of Cultivating Resilience. Psych Central; Psych Central. https://psychcentral.com/lib/mindfulness-the-art-of-cultivating-resilience

Moric, M. (2020, February 5). 5 Types of Power of Attorney Explained. Legal Templates. https://legaltemplates.net/resources/estate-planning/types-of-power-of-attorney/

Nasir, M. (2023, July 5). Importance of Empathy in Healthcare & Caregiving. ConsidraCare. https://www.considracare.com/importance-of-empathy-in-healthcare-caregiving/

Nathan Kobi, (2022, March 30). *Reversible Dementia: Causes, Symptoms, And Treatment.* Geriatric Academy. https://geriatricacademy.com/reversible-causes-of-dementia/

National Family Caregiver Support Program | ACL Administration for Community Living. (2015). Acl.gov. https://acl.gov/programs/support-caregivers/national-family-caregiver-support-program

National Gaucher Foundation. (2020, July 16). 5 Exercises for Building Emotional Resilience | National Gaucher Foundation. National Gaucher Foundation. https://www.gaucherdisease.org/blog/5-exercises-for-building-emotional-resilience/

National Guardianship Association. (2023). Guardianship.org. https://www.guardianship.org/what-is-guardianship/

Osborne, M. (2022, March 3). Care Options For People with Alzheimer's or Other

Dementias | Your Dementia Therapist. Your Dementia Therapist. https://your dementiatherapist.com/alzheimers-dementia/caregiving/options/

Palacio, C., Krikorian, A., María José Gómez-Romero, & Limonero, J. T. (2019). Resilience in Caregivers: A Systematic Review. American Journal of Hospice and Palliative Medicine, 37(8), 648–658. https://doi.org/10.1177/ 1049909119893977

Parkshore Wealth Management. (2022, January 3). Parkshore Wealth Management. https://www.parkshorewealth.com/blog/how-do-you-know-when-its-time-to-put-a-loved-one-in-long-term-care

Patience - The Center for Brain/Mind Medicine. (2022, November 2). The Center for Brain/Mind Medicine. https://cbmm.bwh.harvard.edu/index.php/support-education/for-family-caregivers/patience/#:

Patience when caring. (2018, February 20). Patience when caring for someone living with dementia - NursePartners, Inc. NursePartners, Inc. https://www.nursepartners.org/patience-caring-for-someone-living-with-dementia/

Planning After a Dementia Diagnosis. (2022). Alzheimers.gov. https://www.alzheimers.gov/life-with-dementia/planning-after-diagnosis

Planning Ahead for Legal Matters. (2024). Alzheimer's Disease and Dementia. https://www.alz.org/help-support/caregiving/financial-legal-planning/plan ning-ahead-for-legal-matters

Planning End-of-Life Care for a Person with Dementia and Alzheimers. (2022, April 29). University of Utah Health | University of Utah Health. https://health care.utah.edu/the-scope/health-library/all/2022/04/planning-end-of-life-care-person-dementia-and-alzheimers

Purpose and Types of Guardianship. (2024). Family Law Self-Help Center - Purpose and Types of a Guardianship. Familylawselfhelpcenter.org; Family Law Self-Help Center - Purpose and Types of a Guardianship. https://www.familylawselfhelpcenter.org/self-help/guardianship/overview/purpose-and-types-of-a-guardianship

Ramirez, D. (2023, April 24). Living Trust vs. Will: What's the Difference? NerdWallet. https://www.nerdwallet.com/article/investing/estate-planning/living-trust-vs-will

Reducing caregiver stress. (2022). Alzheimer Society of Canada. https://alzheimer.ca/en/help-support/im-caring-person-living-dementia/looking-after-your self/reducing-caregiver-stress

Robin. (2023). Influence of Sense of Competence, Empathy and Relationship Quality on Burden in Dementia Caregivers: A 15 Months Longitudinal Study - Robin van den Kieboom, Ruth Mark, Liselore Snaphaan, Marcel van Assen, Inge Bongers, 2023. Journal of Applied Gerontology. https://journals.sagepub.com/doi/full/10.1177/07334648221138545

Robinson, L. (2018, November 3). Preventing or Slowing Down Alzheimer's Disease and Dementia. HelpGuide.org. https://www.helpguide.org/articles/alzheimers-dementia-aging/preventing-alzheimers-disease.htm

Samvedna. (2017, September 28). Samvedna Care. Samvednacare.com. https://www.samvednacare.com/blog/empathy-workshop-know-what-it-feels-like-to-be-a-dementia-patient/

Schulz, R., Eden, J., on, C., Board, Health, & and, E. (2016, November 8). Economic Impact of Family Caregiving. Nih.gov; National Academies Press (US). https://www.ncbi.nlm.nih.gov/books/NBK396402/

Sheehan, O. C., Haley, W. E., Howard, V. J., Huang, J., Rhodes, J., & Roth, D. L. (2020). Stress, Burden, and Well-Being in Dementia and Nondementia Caregivers: Insights From the Caregiving Transitions Study. The Gerontologist, 61(5), 670–679. https://doi.org/10.1093/geront/gnaa108

Signs It's Time for Long Term Care - Our Senior Care. (2021, December 13). Our Senior Care. https://ourseniorcare.org/signs-its-time-for-long-term-care/

Smith, M. (2018, October 23). Caregiver Stress and Burnout. HelpGuide.org. https://www.helpguide.org/articles/stress/caregiver-stress-and-burnout.htm

Summerhouse Senior Living. (2023, February 25). Understanding Duties And Responsibilities Of Dementia Caregivers In Houma, LA Memory Care Residences. Summer House Senior Living; Summerhouse Senior Living. https://www.summerhouseseniorliving.com/senior-living-blog/understanding-duties-and-responsibilities-of-dementia-caregivers-in-houma-la-memory-care-residences/

Supported Decision Making - Penn Memory Center. (2023, October 9). Penn Memory Center. https://pennmemorycenter.org/supported-decision-making/

Suzuki, W. (2021, August 31). A neuroscientist shares the 6 exercises she does every day to build resilience and mental strength. CNBC; CNBC. https://www.cnbc.com/2021/08/31/do-these-exercises-every-day-to-build-resilience-and-mental-strength-says-neuroscientist.html

Taking Care of You. (2023). Caregiver.org. https://www.caregiver.org/resource/taking-care-you-self-care-family-caregivers/

The Emotional Side of Caregiving - Family Caregiver Alliance. (2014). Caregiver.org. https://www.caregiver.org/resource/emotional-side-caregiving/

The importance of legal literacy. (2021). Legalliteracyfoundation.com. https://www.legalliteracyfoundation.com/blog/the-importance-of-legal-literacy

The later stage of dementia. (2021, June 18). Alzheimer's Society. https://www.alzheimers.org.uk/about-dementia/symptoms-and-diagnosis/how-dementia-progresses/later-stages-dementia

The later stage of dementia. (2021, June 18). Alzheimer's Society. https://www.

alzheimers.org.uk/about-dementia/symptoms-and-diagnosis/how-dementia-progresses/later-stages-dementia

The middle stage of dementia. (2021, February 24). Alzheimer's Society. https://www.alzheimers.org.uk/about-dementia/symptoms-and-diagnosis/how-dementia-progresses/middle-stage-dementia

The progression, signs and stages of dementia. (2021, February 24). Alzheimer's Society. https://www.alzheimers.org.uk/about-dementia/symptoms-and-diagnosis/how-dementia-progresses/progression-stages-dementia

Three Mindfulness Exercises to Reduce Caregiver Stress. (2017, December 22). Seniors at Home. https://seniorsathome.jfcs.org/mindfulness-exercises-caregivers/

Three real-life stories of dementia, caregiving and communication [YouTube Video]. In YouTube. https://www.youtube.com/watch?v=lbVi_aY_o1Q&t=22s

TIAA Institute. (2023, November). As People Live Longer, Family Caregivers Face Financial Challenges. Prnewswire.com. https://www.prnewswire.com/news-releases/as-people-live-longer-family-caregivers-face-financial-challenges-301970549.html

Trudy. (2021, December 21). Building resilience in caregiving. Ehospice.com. https://ehospice.com/asia-pacific-posts/building-resilience-in-caregiving/

Types of dementia. (2023). Alzheimer's Society. https://www.alzheimers.org.uk/about-dementia/types-dementia

Understand the dementia caregiver's role | Dementia Care Notes. (2010, September 21). Dementia Care Notes, India. https://dementiacarenotes.in/caregivers/understand-caregiving-role/

Understanding Long-Term Care Options for Seniors with Dementia. (2023). Martoncare.com. https://www.martoncare.com/post/long-term-care-dementia

Understanding the Barriers. (2018, November 14). Understanding the Barriers of Dementia Care: Improving Communication and Insight for the Caregiver - Wesbury Retirement Community. Wesbury Retirement Community. https://wesbury.com/2018/11/14/understanding-the-barriers-of-dementia-care-improving-communication-and-insight-for-the-caregiver/

Using Empathy to Care for a Loved One with Alzheimer's. (2019, July 11). Sunrise-seniorliving.com. https://www.sunriseseniorliving.com/resources/dementia-and-memory-care/using-empathy-to-care-for-a-loved-one-with-alzheimers

Using Empathy to Care for a Loved One with Alzheimer's. (2019, July 11). Sunrise-seniorliving.com. https://www.sunriseseniorliving.com/resources/dementia-and-memory-care/using-empathy-to-care-for-a-loved-one-with-alzheimers

Vittayarukskul, L. (2023, September 20). Nine Steps You Can Take in Preparation to Becoming a Caregiver. The Waterlily Blog; The Waterlily Blog. https://blog.

joinwaterlily.com/nine-steps-you-can-take-in-preparation-to-becoming-a-caregiver/

What Are The Main Challenges Faced By Dementia Caregivers? - DementiaWho! (2022, June 11). DementiaWho! https://dementiawho.com/challenges-dementia-caregivers/

What Is Dementia? (2019). Alzheimer's Disease and Dementia. https://www.alz.org/alzheimers-dementia/what-is-dementia

What is Legal Capacity? - Legal Capacity Research. (2017, March 29). Legal Capacity Research - Researching How Mental Capacity Law Works in Everyday Life. https://legalcapacity.org.uk/everyday-decisions/what-is-legal-capacity/

What is vascular dementia? (2022, June 21). Alzheimer's Society. https://www.alzheimers.org.uk/about-dementia/types-dementia/vascular-dementia

Zarko, J. (2018). *The caregiver perspective: Jennifer's story*. https://blogs.ohsu.edu/brain/2018/03/23/the-caregiver-perspective-jennifers-story/

www.ingramcontent.com/pod-product-compliance
Lightning Source LLC
Chambersburg PA
CBHW022052020426
42335CB00012B/656